Interventional Radiological Treatment of Liver Tumors

Contemporary Issues in Cancer Imaging

A Multidisciplinary Approach

Series Editor

Rodney H. Reznek

Cancer Imaging, St Bartholomew's Hospital, London

Editorial Adviser

Janet E. Husband

Diagnostic Radiology, Royal Marsden Hospital, Surrey

Current titles in the series

Cancer of the Ovary
Lung Cancer
Colorectal Cancer
Carcinoma of the Kidney
Carcinoma of the Esophagus
Carcinoma of the Bladder
Prostate Cancer
Squamous Cell Cancer of the Neck

Forthcoming titles in the series

Pancreatic Cancer
Gastric Cancer
Primary Carcinomas of the Liver
Breast Cancer

Interventional Radiological Treatment of Liver Tumors

Edited by

Andy Adam

Peter R. Mueller

Series Editor

Rodney H. Reznek

Editorial Adviser

Janet E. Husband

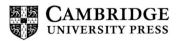
CAMBRIDGE
UNIVERSITY PRESS

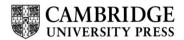

CAMBRIDGE
UNIVERSITY PRESS

Shaftesbury Road, Cambridge CB2 8EA, United Kingdom

One Liberty Plaza, 20th Floor, New York, NY 10006, USA

477 Williamstown Road, Port Melbourne, VIC 3207, Australia

314–321, 3rd Floor, Plot 3, Splendor Forum, Jasola District Centre, New Delhi – 110025, India

103 Penang Road, #05–06/07, Visioncrest Commercial, Singapore 238467

Cambridge University Press is part of Cambridge University Press & Assessment,
a department of the University of Cambridge.

We share the University's mission to contribute to society through the pursuit of
education, learning and research at the highest international levels of excellence.

www.cambridge.org
Information on this title: www.cambridge.org/9780521886871

First published 2009

A catalogue record for this publication is available from the British Library

ISBN   978-0-521-88687-1   Hardback

Cambridge University Press & Assessment has no responsibility for the persistence
or accuracy of URLs for external or third-party internet websites referred to in this
publication and does not guarantee that any content on such websites is, or will
remain, accurate or appropriate.

....

Every effort has been made in preparing this book to provide accurate and up-to-date
information which is in accord with accepted standards and practice at the time of
publication. Although case histories are drawn from actual cases, every effort has been
made to disguise the identities of the individuals involved. Nevertheless, the authors,
editors and publishers can make no warranties that the information contained herein
is totally free from error, not least because clinical standards are constantly changing
through research and regulation. The authors, editors and publishers therefore
disclaim all liability for direct or consequential damages resulting from the use of
material contained in this book. Readers are strongly advised to pay careful attention
to information provided by the manufacturer of any drugs or equipment that they plan
to use.

Contents

Color plate section appears between pages 50 and 51.

Contributors

Gregory Avey
Department of Radiology
University of Wisconsin
Madison, Wisconsin, USA

Kambadakone R. Avinssh
Department of Radiology
Massachusetts General Hospital
Harvard Medical School
Boston, Massachusetts, USA

Elena Bozzi
Resident in Radiology
Department of Oncology Transplants and
Advanced Technologies in Medicine
University of Pisa
Pisa, Italy

Dania Cioni
Assistant Professor of Radiology
Department of Oncology Transplants and
Advanced Technologies in Medicine
University of Pisa
Pisa, Italy

Laura Crocetti
Assistant Professor of Radiology
Department of Oncology Transplants and
Advanced Technologies in Medicine
University of Pisa
Pisa, Italy

Gerald D. Dodd, III
Professor and Chair
Liver Tumor Ablation Service
Department of Radiology
University of Texas Health Science Center at
San Antonio
San Antonio, Texas, USA

Fadi M. El-Merhi
Assistant Professor
Liver Tumor Ablation Service
Department of Radiology
University of Texas Health Science Center at
San Antonio
San Antonio, Texas, USA

Yuman Fong
Murray F. Brennan Chair in Surgery
Memorial Sloan-Kettering Cancer Center
New York, New York, USA

Suvranu Ganguli
Laboratory for Minimally Invasive Tumor
Therapy
Department of Radiology
Beth Israel Deaconess Medical Center
Harvard Medical School
Boston, Massachusetts, USA

S. Nahum Goldberg
Laboratory for Minimally Invasive Tumor
Therapy
Department of Radiology
Beth Israel Deaconess Medical Center
Harvard Medical School
Boston, Massachusetts, USA

Debra A. Gervais
Department of Radiology
Massachusetts General Hospital
Harvard Medical School
Boston, Massachusetts, USA

J. Louis Hinshaw
Department of Radiology
University of Wisconsin
Madison, Wisconsin, USA

C. S. Ho
Professor and Consultant Radiologist
University of Toronto
University Health Network and
Mt Sinai Hospital
Department of Medical Imaging
Toronto, Ontario, Canada

Linda G. Hubbard
Nurse Coordinator
Liver Tumor Ablation Service
Department of Radiology
University of Texas Health Science Center at
San Antonio
San Antonio, Texas, USA

Chaturika Jayadewa
Joint Physics Department
Royal Marsden Hospital
Sutton, Surrey, UK

Philip Johnson
Cancer Research UK Institute for Cancer Studies
University of Birmingham
Birmingham, UK

Masamichi Kojiro
Department of Pathology
Kurume University School of Medicine
Kurume, Japan

Troy Kimsey
Surgical Oncology Fellow
Memorial Sloan-Kettering Cancer Center
New York, New York, USA

Fred T. Lee Jr.
Department of Radiology
University of Wisconsin
Madison, Wisconsin, USA

Riccardo Lencioni
Associate Professor of Radiology
Department of Oncology Transplants and
Advanced Technologies in Medicine
University of Pisa
Pisa, Italy

Chang-Hsien Liu
Department of Radiology
Massachusetts General Hospital
Harvard Medical School
Boston, Massachusetts, USA *and*
Department of Radiology
Tri-Service General Hospital and National
Defense Medical Center
Taipei, Taiwan

Daniel Palmer
Cancer Research UK Institute for Cancer Studies
University of Birmingham
Birmingham, UK

Alexander T. Ruutiainen
Dept of Radiology
Hospital of the University of Pennsylvania
Philadelphia, Pennsylvania, USA

Dushyant V. Sahani
Associate Professor of Radiology
Department of Radiology
Massachusetts General Hospital
Harvard Medical School
Boston, Massachusetts, USA

Michael Soulen
Dept of Radiology
Hospital of the University of Pennsylvania
Philadelphia, Pennsylvania, USA

K. T. Tan
Assistant Professor and Staff Radiologist
University of Toronto
University Health Network and
Mt Sinai Hospital
Department of Medical Imaging
Toronto, Ontario, Canada

Gail ter Haar
Joint Physics Department
Royal Marsden Hospital
Sutton, Surrey, UK

Sadaf Zahur
Joint Physics Department
Royal Marsden Hospital
Sutton, Surrey, UK

Series foreword

Imaging has become pivotal in all aspects of the management of patients with cancer. At the same time, it is acknowledged that optimal patient care is best achieved by a multidisciplinary team approach. The explosion of technological developments in imaging over the past years has meant that all members of the multidisciplinary team should understand the potential applications, limitations, and advantages of all the evolving and exciting imaging techniques. Equally, to understand the significance of the imaging findings and to contribute actively to management decisions and to the development of new clinical applications for imaging, it is critical that the radiologist should have sufficient background knowledge of different tumors. Thus the radiologist should understand the pathology, the clinical background, the therapeutic options, and prognostic indicators of malignancy.

Contemporary Issues in Cancer Imaging – A Multidisciplinary Approach aims to meet the growing requirement for radiologists to have detailed knowledge of the individual tumors in which they are involved in making management decisions. A series of single-subject issues, each of which will be dedicated to a single tumor site, edited by recognized expert guest editors, will include contributions from basic scientists, pathologists, surgeons, oncologists, radiologists, and others.

While the series is written predominantly for the radiologist, it is hoped that individual issues will contain sufficiently varied information so as to be of interest to all medical disciplines and to other health professionals managing patients with cancer. As with imaging, advances have occurred in all these disciplines related to cancer management, and it is our fervent hope that this series, bringing together expertise from such a range of related specialties, will not only promote the understanding and rational application of modern imaging but will also help to achieve the ultimate goal of improving outcomes for patients with cancer.

Rodney H. Reznek

Preface to Interventional Radiological Treatment of Liver Tumors

The care of patients with malignant tumors has changed substantially in recent years. New chemotherapeutic agents have led to substantial prolongation of survival in patients with liver metastases. Advances in surgery and anesthesia have enabled the resection of tumors with much lower morbidity and mortality. Diagnostic imaging techniques have facilitated earlier detection and more detailed follow-up of patients with liver tumors. However, the most exciting advances have been in the field of interventional radiology. Percutaneous ethanol injection, which has been used most effectively and extensively in the Far East, demonstrated that it is possible to completely destroy small hepatocellular carcinomas, obviating the need for surgical removal. This paved the way for the development of other local methods of treatment based on heating or freezing malignant tumors.

This book describes the state of the art in one of the most exciting fields in modern medicine. The authors are all world authorities in their field. The volume focuses on interventional radiological techniques but also provides a summary of the pathology of liver tumors, as well as an account of modern medical and surgical methods of treatment.

We are still in the early stages of local tumor treatment. The early results are very promising, and it is very likely that, in time, traditional surgical techniques will be increasingly supplemented by image-guided methods. Coupled with advances in structural and functional imaging, these advances offer the hope that a substantial proportion of patients with hepatic malignancy can be treated effectively.

Andy Adam and
Peter R. Mueller

1

The clinical management of hepatic neoplasms

Daniel Palmer and Philip Johnson

Introduction

The liver is the organ most frequently involved by cancer. In developing countries hepatocellular carcinoma is a major public health problem responsible for over 500 000 deaths per year [1]. In the West its incidence is rising, in part due to the increasing prevalence of chronic hepatitis C virus infection [2,3]. The liver is also the commonest site of metastases, and up to 75% of primary tumors drained by the portal venous system involve the liver before death.

This chapter will review the epidemiology, etiology, and current management of hepatocellular carcinoma and of secondary liver cancer, with particular reference to colorectal metastases as a paradigm for the multidisciplinary management of cancer.

Hepatocellular carcinoma

Epidemiology and etiology

Hepatocellular carcinoma (HCC) is one of the commonest malignancies world-wide but with wide geographical variation, the highest incidence occurring in sub-Saharan Africa and the Far East [1]. This variation suggests the importance of environmental factors (Table 1.1). Prime among these are chronic infection by hepatitis viruses B and C (HBV and HCV) and exposure to aflatoxin. In a study of 22 000 Chinese males, 15% of whom were HBV carriers, the relative risk for HCC development in HBV-positive men was 98.4 [4]. An HBV vaccination program, inoculating neonates, was initiated in Taiwan in the early 1980s and has resulted in a clear reduction in the incidence of childhood HCC [5]. However, an effect on the incidence of HCC in adults may take a further 20 years to become apparent. Evidence also suggests that genotype Ce is an important risk factor, and antiviral

Interventional Radiological Treatment of Liver Tumors, ed. Andy Adam and Peter R. Mueller.
Published by Cambridge University Press. © Cambridge University Press 2009.

Table 1.1 Major risk factors for hepatocellular carcinoma

Chronic liver disease (usually at the stage of cirrhosis)
Chronic hepatitis B virus infection
Chronic hepatitis C virus infection
Dietary exposure to aflatoxin
Increasing age
Male gender

therapy in patients with chronic hepatitis B may also reduce the incidence of HCC [6,7]. The epidemiological evidence linking chronic HCV infection and HCC is similar to that for HBV. In a study of almost 10 000 Chinese males, 5% of whom were HCV-positive, the relative risk for HCC was 21.5 [8]. Although there is no vaccine against HCV there is increasing evidence that a sustained virological response to interferon or interferon/ribavirin decreases the risk of HCC development, while the 1b genotype increases it [9,10]. The great majority of HCCs arise in the setting of chronic liver disease, usually at the stage of cirrhosis, and all types of cirrhosis, particularly in males, are at a high risk of developing HCC [11].

Aflatoxin, produced by the fungus *Aspergillus flavus*, which grows on cereals stored in damp conditions, is one of the most potent liver carcinogens known, and a clear relationship between intake and incidence of HCC exists in high HCC incidence areas. As well as methods to improve grain storage to reduce aflatoxin exposure, the possibility of chemoprevention is an area of active research [12,13].

Diagnosis

The functional reserve of the liver is such that tumors can reach a considerable size before causing symptoms or signs, typically right upper quadrant pain, hepatomegaly, and weight loss. Decompensation of chronic liver disease (variceal hemorrhage, ascites, encephalopathy) is also a frequent presentation. Less commonly, a tumor may rupture, resulting in severe abdominal pain, shock, and hemoperitoneum [14]. Rarer presentations include hypoglycemia, hypercalcemia, and polycythemia due to tumor secretion of insulin-like growth factors, parathyroid-related hormones, and erythropoietin, respectively [15]. HCC is increasingly diagnosed pre-symptomatically as a result of screening programs.

Dynamic triphasic computed tomography (CT) or gadolinium-enhanced magnetic resonance imaging (MRI) will classically show marked enhancement in the arterial phase with relative hypovascularity ("washout") in the portal or late phases. The European Association for the Study of the Liver (EASL) criteria state that in a patient with cirrhosis and a mass greater than 2 cm, this radiological appearance (confirmed by two imaging modalities) is diagnostic of HCC without the need for histology [16]. The presence of an enhancing liver mass on one imaging modality with a serum alpha-fetoprotein (AFP) level greater than 400 ng mL^{-1} is also considered diagnostic.

Cross-sectional imaging is required to stage the disease so that treatment can be planned. In particular, size, number, and distribution of tumors can be established, as well as the presence of macrovascular (portal vein) invasion and extra-hepatic disease. Although contrast-enhanced CT and MRI are the best current imaging modalities, both techniques may miss up to 30% of lesions (as detected in the explanted liver following liver transplantation), especially those less than 1 cm [17].

Serum AFP is elevated in 70% of patients with HCC [18]. It is of value in the diagnosis of HCC in patients with cirrhosis and has been used as a surveillance tool in high-risk populations. However, levels of 500 ng mL^{-1} or more can occur in benign liver diseases, notably chronic active hepatitis and fulminant liver failure. Nevertheless, a rising AFP is strongly suggestive of HCC. It may also be useful in monitoring the effects of treatment and for the detection of disease recurrence or progression following treatment.

For a liver mass not fulfilling the EASL criteria, a diagnosis of HCC requires histological confirmation. Fine-needle biopsy may be limited by sampling error, particularly for small lesions, and by difficulty in distinguishing well-differentiated HCC from dysplasia or adenoma. Some groups believe that biopsy may risk tumor seeding along the needle track and recommend avoidance of the procedure in candidates for surgical resection or transplantation. Histological type is not of prognostic significance, with the exception of the fibrolamellar variant, which typically occurs in younger patients without underlying chronic liver disease. In this setting, resection rates are higher and prognosis is better (median survival 5 years), although this may reflect the younger age and absence of cirrhosis [19].

Screening

Since HCC predominantly occurs on the background of chronic liver disease, usually at the stage of cirrhosis, this has a significant impact on the mode of presentation, complicates diagnosis, and limits therapeutic options. Thus, the identification of risk factors (Table 1.1), which may lead to interventions that reduce its incidence and form the basis of screening programs for high-risk populations, is of particular importance. There is some evidence that this can reduce disease-specific mortality [20]. Current guidelines suggest that those in a high-risk group undergo 6-monthly ultrasound examinations. Serial AFP measurement has limited sensitivity, and whether or not it should be used as a part of a screening program remains controversial [21–23].

Staging and prognosis

For most cancers, prognosis is predominantly determined by tumor stage. However, HCCs usually occur on a background of cirrhosis, which independently contributes to prognosis [24]. For the majority of patients, prognosis is poor, with treatments other than surgery having little impact on survival. Tumor size is a key prognostic factor, with survival approaching 3 years for tumors less than 3 cm but only 3 months for those larger than 8 cm [25]. Vascular invasion increases with tumor size, but is an independent prognostic factor; even large tumors can have a good prognosis following surgical resection in the absence of vascular invasion [26,27]. Underlying cirrhosis may limit prognosis and can influence treatment options such as surgical resection and chemoembolization, which require sufficient hepatic reserve to be performed safely. Prognostic models for HCC are therefore complex and should take into account tumor stage, degree of liver impairment, patient fitness, and treatment efficacy.

Treatment options for HCC

Liver resection

The ability to resect a tumor depends on its size, location, relation to blood vessels, and underlying liver function. In patients without cirrhosis, up to 75% of the liver can be removed safely, and hepatic resection is the treatment of choice. Resection in patients with cirrhosis is still associated with significant morbidity and mortality, although this has fallen to less than 5% with recognition of the segmental anatomy of the liver, improvements in surgical technique and postoperative management, combined with better patient selection. Less than 20% of patients are suitable for resection, although this may increase as screening programs detect tumors at an earlier stage. Survival is better for solitary tumors less than 5 cm with negative resection margins and an absence of vascular invasion or lymph-node involvement, with 5-year survival up to 70% [28,29].

Table 1.2 Eligibility criteria for liver transplantation in patients with hepatocellular carcinoma

Milan criteria	UCSF criteria
One tumor < 5 cm	One tumor < 6.5 cm
or	*or*
Up to 3 nodules, each ≤ 3 cm	Up to 3 nodules, each ≤ 4.5 cm, and total tumor diameter ≤ 8 cm

Transplantation

Liver transplantation has the potential to treat both tumor and underlying cirrhosis, although patients with viral hepatitis have a risk of reinfection in the new liver. Assessment of tumor size and number, vascular involvement, and extrahepatic disease is essential to identify those patients most likely to benefit. In patients with no more than three tumors less than 5 cm, survival is similar to that of patients with benign end-stage liver disease, and, where available, transplantation is the treatment of choice for HCC in a cirrhotic liver. This experience has led to the development of the Milan criteria (Table 1.2) to guide the selection of patients for transplantation, which can lead to 5-year survival in excess of 70% [30]. Recent reports indicate that these criteria may be extended whilst retaining good outcomes (University of California San Francisco criteria, Table 1.2) [31].

A major limitation to transplantation is the supply of donor organs. This results in a period, of uncertain duration, between listing and transplantation, with the risk that the tumor will grow beyond the criteria for transplant [32]. Thus, scoring systems used to allocate donor organs are weighted to prioritize patients with HCC [33]. Drop-out (disease progression to a level at which transplantation is no longer appropriate whilst awaiting a donor liver) may be best reduced by increasing the number/availability of donor organs, and this may be helped by the use of living donors. Early data indicate similar results to those achieved with cadaveric organs if the Milan criteria are followed, with low mortality amongst donors [34].

Many centers employ treatments such as local ablation and chemoembolization (see below) to bridge the gap between listing and receipt of the transplant, although there are no prospective randomized data to indicate the utility of this strategy [35].

Local ablation

Ablative therapies, including percutaneous ethanol injection and thermal ablation, appear, by many criteria, to be as effective as surgery in appropriately selected cases. Like surgery, however, they are less effective as tumor size increases, particularly beyond 5 cm. As well as increasing difficulty in achieving complete ablation, this probably reflects the fact that as tumors increase in size the frequency of vascular invasion increases and, with it, the likelihood of metastasis.

Treatment is usually performed percutaneously under image guidance. Several methods for tumor destruction have been used, the most widely studied being percutaneous ethanol injection (PEI) and radiofrequency ablation (RFA). Injection of 90% ethanol under ultrasound guidance is technically straightforward, inexpensive, safe, and, depending on the severity of underlying cirrhosis, can result in 5-year survival of up to 50% [36]. Complete tumor necrosis is achieved in 70% of tumors less than 3 cm in diameter, but this falls with increasing size, probably due to the inability of the injected volume to disperse evenly throughout larger tumors.

Radiofrequency ablation is a localized thermal treatment producing tumor destruction by heating a probe inserted into the tumor to temperatures exceeding 60 °C, which can be performed percutaneously under image guidance, laparoscopically, or at laparotomy. The procedure is of limited applicability for subcapsular lesions, and when a large blood vessel is nearby it is difficult to obtain sufficiently high temperatures for complete tumor necrosis because of the heat-sink effect.

Randomized studies have compared RFA with PEI. A study in patients with tumors up to 4 cm demonstrated that RFA was superior in terms of tumor necrosis and survival, with 3-year survival of 74% versus 51% [37]. Further studies have demonstrated similar advantages for RFA in treating smaller tumors [38,39]. In general, RFA was associated with fewer sessions to achieve complete tumor necrosis, with no significant differences in morbidity and a likely improvement in survival.

Transarterial chemoembolization

HCC is a highly vascularized tumor, mostly via the hepatic artery. In contrast, nontumorous liver parenchyma derives most of its blood supply from the portal vein. Thus, transarterial chemoembolization (TACE) utilizes selective catheterization of the hepatic artery to deliver regional chemotherapy and embolize tumor-feeding arteries (Fig. 1.1). Chemotherapy is first injected, often mixed with lipiodol, an oily compound that accumulates preferentially in tumors, probably via enhanced permeability of

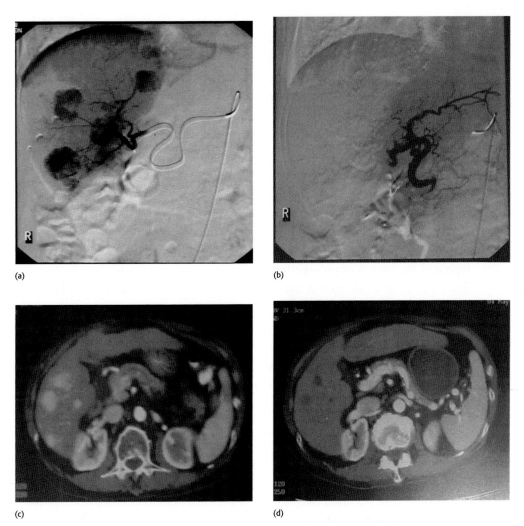

(a)   (b)

(c)   (d)

Figure 1.1 Transarterial chemoembolization. (a, b) Hepatic arterial angiography. (c, d) Contrast-enhanced CT. Pre-embolization (a and c) demonstrating hypervascular multifocal HCC. Post-embolization (b and d) showing tumor circulation abolished. *See color plate section.*

leaky tumor vasculature and retention due to impaired lymphatic drainage, with the aim of retaining the chemotherapy to increase tumor concentration and reduce systemic exposure. This is followed by embolization of tumor-feeding arteries using one of a variety of embolic materials [40,41]. For chemoembolization to be performed safely, there must be adequate blood supply to the non-tumorous liver via the portal vein, and it is therefore contraindicated in the presence of main portal vein thrombosis. Other contraindications include extrahepatic disease, advanced cirrhosis, and poor performance status. Embolization is frequently complicated by a characteristic syndrome of abdominal pain, fever, and nausea, which is normally self-limiting within 2–4 days, although occasionally patients go on to develop liver abscess [42].

Two recent randomized controlled trials and a meta-analysis have demonstrated a survival benefit for patients receiving TACE compared with supportive care [43–45]. The general applicability of these data is limited by the relatively small sample size, and by the heterogeneity of the patient populations and the techniques used, with differences in the choice of chemotherapeutic agent, embolic agent, and use of lipiodol. Nevertheless, the key to successful chemoembolization is undoubtedly patient selection, and both the positive trials suggest the ideal candidate has well-preserved liver function and asymptomatic disease.

A major limitation of locoregional approaches is disease recurrence, which may represent the growth of pre-existing micrometastases from the primary tumor or the development of a new tumor, considered, arbitrarily, to have occurred when tumor develops more than 3 years after treatment. Since local recurrence may reflect pre-existing micrometastases in the immediate vicinity of the primary tumor, the ability of RFA to achieve a wider margin may explain its superiority to PEI.

In the absence of an effective systemic agent, there are no conclusive data that adjuvant treatment can decrease the risk of tumor recurrence.

Systemic therapies for HCC

The majority of patients with HCC have multifocal disease, bilobar disease, extrahepatic disease, and/or underlying cirrhosis, such that surgery, ablation, or chemoembolization are not indicated. For these patients, systemic therapy is required.

Chemotherapy

Objective radiological response rates for single-agent chemotherapy are low. The most widely used drug has been doxorubicin, although systematic reviews of randomized trials have failed to discern a significant survival benefit [46]. Combination chemotherapy can induce higher response rates in the range of 20–30%, but with no evidence of a significant impact on survival [47].

Interpretation of the impact of chemotherapy is limited by the small size of clinical trials and the heterogenous patient groups. More recently, a large-scale trial has investigated the novel thymidylate synthase inhibitor nolatrexed, using doxorubicin as the comparator. Despite encouraging evidence of activity in earlier-phase trials, in fact patients receiving nolatrexed survived for a significantly shorter time than those in the control arm (4.7 compared to 6.9 months, $p = 0.0068$). Whilst the statistical assumptions used in the design of this trial were based on demonstrating superiority for nolatrexed, since there were no obvious nolatrexed-related early deaths some have argued that this study provides evidence that doxorubicin may, in fact, positively influence survival in appropriately selected patients [48]. Nevertheless, whilst conventional cytotoxic therapy has undoubted activity against HCC, whether or not this translates into a survival advantage has still not been rigorously demonstrated [49].

Endocrine therapies have been investigated in HCC based on reports of estrogen receptor expression in some cases. Early small studies with anti-estrogenic and anti-androgenic agents showed promise [50]. However, large prospective controlled studies have refuted any role for hormonal agents including tamoxifen [51].

Octreotide, a somatostatin analogue used to treat carcinoid tumors by suppressing the secretion of peptide hormones, has been tested in HCC based on proposed suppression of tropic hormones (insulin and insulin-like growth factors), anti-angiogenic activity, and presence of somatostatin receptors on HCC [52,53]. However, whilst an initial small study suggested promising activity, this has not been corroborated in subsequent larger randomized trials [54–56].

Angiogenesis and hepatocellular carcinoma

As a tumor grows to exceed the size at which oxygen enters by diffusion, development of a blood supply is essential. Vascular endothelial growth factor (VEGF) is a key signaling protein involved in angiogenesis, acting predominantly on vascular endothelial cells via VEGF receptor 2. VEGF production is stimulated by hypoxia, and circulating VEGF then binds to its receptors on endothelial cells, triggering a tyrosine kinase signaling cascade leading to upregulation of genes that promote angiogenesis. In HCC there is overexpression of VEGF, which appears to correlate with the degree of differentiation and tumor size [57,58]. Angiogenesis can be inhibited pharmacologically either by small molecule inhibitors of VEGF receptor signaling (e.g., sorafenib) or through a monoclonal antibody targeted against VEGF preventing its interaction with receptors (e.g., bevacizumab). Both approaches have entered clinical trials in patients with HCC.

Sorafenib

Sorafenib is an oral multikinase inhibitor that targets the Raf/MEK/ERK growth-factor signaling pathway, which has increased activity in HCC [59]. A molecular abnormality common to many human cancers, including HCC, is abnormal growth-factor receptor signaling such that growth signals may be constitutively activated independently of the growth factor itself, resulting in uncontrolled cell proliferation and survival. In the active form, growth-factor receptors stimulate a signaling cascade in the cell cytoplasm whereby a series of enzymes is activated, often by phosphorylation. This cascade allows amplification and diversification of the signal. The Raf/MEK/ERK signaling pathway is one of those downstream of growth-factor receptors, and thus its inhibition may inhibit the deregulated growth of malignant cells (Fig. 1.2).

Sorafenib also targets VEGF receptor tyrosine kinases. Thus, sorafenib has direct anti-tumor and anti-angiogenic properties. In a phase II study, whilst the objective

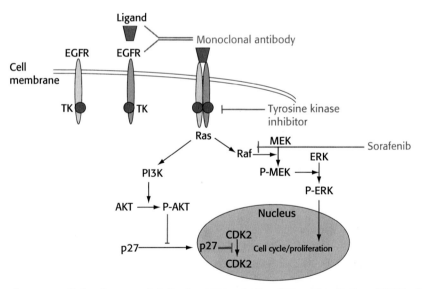

Figure 1.2 **Cell signaling cascade following EGFR activation. Heterodimerization of EGFR with other HER receptors activates Ras, which activates PI3K to promote phosphorylation of AKT. Phosphorylated AKT inhibits nuclear translocation of p27, resulting in the loss of its inhibitory effect on cyclin dependent kinase 2 (CDK2). This allows CDK2 to promote entry into cell cycle with resultant cell proliferation. This growth stimulatory pathway can be inhibited at the level of the EGFR receptor (e.g., cetuximab), by inhibition of EGF receptor tyrosine kinase activity (e.g., erlotinib), or by inhibitors acting downstream of Akt (e.g., m-Tor inhibitors). Ras also activates the Raf/MEK/ERK pathway to promote cell proliferation, a process that can be inhibited by sorafenib.**

response rate was very low (2.2%), a disease stability rate of 33% at 4 months and median survival of 9 months were seen as sufficiently encouraging to proceed to a large randomized placebo-controlled trial [60]. Six hundred and two patients were randomly assigned either sorafenib or placebo. Patients were predominantly European, with Child A cirrhosis and good performance status. Treatment was well tolerated with diarrhoea, fatigue, and skin toxicity being the most commonly reported side effects. Sorafenib was associated with a significant improvement in overall survival compared to placebo (median survival 10.7 vs. 7.9 months, $p = 0.00007$) [61]. Although sorafenib is the first systemic agent to clearly demonstrate a survival advantage in patients with HCC, other novel agents are showing promise in early-phase trials.

Sunitinib is another multikinase inhibitor targeting VEGF and PDGF receptor tyrosine kinases. Phase II data are similar to sorafenib, and phase III trials are planned [62]. Bevacizumab is a humanized murine anti-VEGF monoclonal antibody, which in combination with cytotoxic chemotherapy has shown activity in metastatic colorectal carcinoma (see below). Phase II studies in patients with HCC have indicated modest activity [63].

Tumor angiogenesis is regulated predominantly, but not exclusively, through VEGF signaling. The epidermal growth factor (EGF) and transforming growth factor alpha (TGFα) play a major role in angiogenesis, and in cancer cell proliferation and invasion. Both are active through the EGF receptor, which is commonly overexpressed in HCC (Fig. 1.2) [64]. Erlotinib is an orally active inhibitor of EGFR tyrosine kinase. Phase II studies have reported partial responses and encouraging disease stabilization in HCC [65,66].

The complexity and redundancy within tumor cell and endothelial cell signaling suggests that inhibition of one single pathway is unlikely to meet with dramatic success. Increased understanding of these processes does provide evidence for the rational combination of several agents, and such combinations are now entering clinical trials. For example, there is laboratory evidence of synergy between VEGF and EGF inhibition. The promising results for bevacizumab and erlotinib used singly has led to investigation of their use in combination, with encouraging results from a phase II study reporting a response rate of 22% and 55% progression-free survival at 16 weeks [67]. A phase III study comparing this combination with sorafenib is planned.

Pathways that are inhibited by novel targeted therapies, including Raf/MEK/ERK, may also contribute to resistance to conventional chemotherapeutic agents, and combination of these agents with chemotherapy may overcome chemoresistance. A randomized phase II study has addressed this question by combining sorafenib with systemic doxorubicin. Combination therapy was well tolerated and was associated with a significant prolongation of overall survival compared to doxorubicin alone (13.7 vs. 6.5 months, $p = 0.049$) [68]. To establish whether this benefit is attributable to synergy between the two agents or to sorafenib alone requires a further randomized trial of the combination using sorafenib as the control arm.

With the plethora of agents and combinations that are becoming available, decisions about which agents should progress to large-scale phase III trials must be made. Traditionally, for conventional chemotherapy, radiological response has been the preferred end point for phase II trials. However, many newer agents may not cause tumor shrinkage but rather disease stabilization, and this requires novel trial design incorporating, for example, time to progression or progression-free survival end points, necessitating serial radiological assessments.

A critical challenge in the development of these therapies is the incorporation of translational research end points into clinical trial design in order to identify the presence of the relevant target in the tumor and to correlate this with response so that patients most likely to benefit can be selected.

Radiation therapy

The use of external-beam radiotherapy is significantly limited by the radiosensitivity of normal hepatocytes, with normal tissue tolerance 25–30 Gy and higher doses increasing the risk of radiation hepatitis [69]. Conformal techniques allow tumor doses up to 72 Gy without severe hepatitis and with objective responses [70]. Radioisotopes can be delivered via the hepatic artery using yttrium-90-labeled microspheres or iodine-131-containing lipiodol. Iodine-131 lipiodol, a gamma emitter, can induce response rates of 40%, whilst limiting radiation dose to normal liver to less than 20 Gy [71]. Yttrium-90 is a beta emitter with shorter tissue penetration, which may further improve normal liver tolerance and reduce the risk of radiation hepatitis [72]. Radioembolization is associated with a risk of lung toxicity if there is extensive arteriovenous shunting in patients with cirrhosis, and an assessment of the degree of shunting is required prior to treatment. Further, precise and laborious angiographic mapping is essential, to define any aberrant vascular anatomy (which may be particularly common from the left hepatic artery) and avoid radioembolization of the GI tract. To date the impact on survival has not been defined.

Management of colorectal liver metastases

In colorectal cancer (CRC) the liver is frequently the sole or predominant site of metastatic disease. Untreated, median survival for patients with liver metastases is 6 months. However, in carefully selected patients local treatment is potentially curative. Recent advances in cytotoxic chemotherapy also introduce the possibility of downstaging liver metastases, extending the limits of resectability.

Surgical resection of liver metastases

The initial investigation of suspected liver metastases is either CT or MRI scan. In terms of assessment of suitability for resection both have a sensitivity and specificity of 90% [73]. PET scanning is increasingly used in those potentially suitable for resection, as it may detect previously undiagnosed extrahepatic disease. Whilst extrahepatic disease is usually a contraindication, occasionally surgery can be successful, for example in resecting solitary lung metastases.

In 20% of patients with colorectal cancer, liver metastases are present at the same time as the primary lesion presents (synchronous), and a further 50% will eventually develop metastases (metachronous). Of these, complete surgical resection is feasible in less than 20% [74,75]. Patients with liver-predominant disease should be referred to a hepatobiliary multidisciplinary team for consideration of resection. If complete resection with clear surgical margins can be achieved, long-term survival can be expected in 30–50% of patients. Preoperative embolization of the portal vein branches supplying the lobe of liver to be resected can expand the volume of the remnant, which may allow extended liver resections if required.

Radiofrequency ablation for liver metastases

The integration of ablative therapies may further expand the number of patients eligible for potentially curative treatment. Retrospective series suggest a survival benefit for patients with colorectal liver metastases treated by RFA (median survival 30–36 months) compared with historical controls. Indeed, some groups suggest that RFA may be equivalent to surgery in treating small-volume disease [76]. RFA is also commonly used intraoperatively for patients undergoing liver resection, to treat additional lesions not incorporated within the field of resection.

To date, there are no prospective randomized trials to clearly define the most appropriate application of RFA in the management of colorectal liver metastases.

However, trials randomly assigning patients either between surgery and RFA or between systemic chemotherapy and RFA are difficult to conduct in terms of acceptability to patients because of the radical differences between the treatment modalities.

Systemic therapy for colorectal cancer

In patients with colorectal cancer, chemotherapy is used for metastatic disease to palliate symptoms and prolong survival. In some cases, this may result in "down-staging" liver metastases so that resection may be possible. Chemotherapy may also be used as an adjuvant following surgery to remove the primary tumor, with the aim of reducing the risk of recurrence.

The backbone of chemotherapy for CRC remains 5-fluorouracil (5-FU), a drug that was rationally designed in the 1950s to interfere with DNA and RNA synthesis through inhibition of the enzyme thymidylate synthase (TS) [77].

Recent advances have resulted in modest increments in survival, primarily due to the introduction of new cytotoxic and biological agents but partly due to the development of more sophisticated radiological techniques that allow the diagnosis of liver metastases earlier, often while the patient is asymptomatic, making for an apparent increase in survival.

Capecitabine is a fluoropyrimidine precursor that is converted to 5-FU by a series of enzymatic reactions. Unlike 5-FU, its oral bioavailability is predictable. It appears to be at least as effective as 5-FU, but avoids the need for infusion pumps and venous access [78]. Capecitabine can probably substitute for 5-FU in combination regimens. Irinotecan inhibits topoisomerase I, a DNA-unwinding enzyme required for cell division. It first demonstrated improved survival as a single agent compared to supportive care in patients with 5-FU-refractory disease [79]. Randomized studies have shown that when irinotecan is added to 5-FU as a first-line treatment there is an increase in median survival of 3 months compared to 5-FU alone at the expense of increased toxicity including diarrhoea, vomiting, abdominal cramping, and vascular complications (acute myocardial infarction, pulmonary embolus, and cerebrovascular accident) [80–82]. When irinotecan was administered in combination with bolus 5-FU, fatal toxicity was as high as 5% compared to less than 1% in the control (5-FU) arm. Combination with infusional 5-FU appears to be more tolerable.

Oxaliplatin is a diaminocylcohexane platinum derivative with a different spectrum of activity from the widely used cisplatin and carboplatin. It also has a different spectrum of toxicity, with no renal toxicity but marked neurological toxicity characterized by a sensory peripheral neuropathy, which is cumulative but largely reversible upon discontinuation of treatment. In preclinical models there was activity against colon cancer cell lines and synergy with 5-FU. Phase II trials reported a 10–25% response rate when oxaliplatin was used as a single agent in metastatic colorectal cancer, but 50% in combination with 5-FU [83]. Randomized trials of oxaliplatin with 5-FU confirmed the high response rate, but improvement in overall survival was not achieved, in part due to crossover, where a significant number of patients initially assigned to 5-FU alone received oxaliplatin upon progression [84]. Subsequently, oxaliplatin combined with 5-FU has shown equivalent activity to irinotecan-based regimens, and 5-FU combined with either oxaliplatin or irinotecan can be considered equivalent first-line treatments [85,86].

With three active chemotherapy agents available for the palliation of advanced CRC, choices must be made regarding sequencing and duration of treatment. The decision process takes into account the objectives of treatment, the extent of disease and its associated symptoms, comorbid conditions, the likely side-effect profile, and patient preferences. In general, oxaliplatin combined with a fluoropyrimidine (either capecitabine or 5-FU) constitutes a common first-line combination followed by irinotecan (alone or in combination with fluoropyrimidine) as second-line treatment providing performance status remains adequate. This decision may be influenced by the potential toxicity profile. For example, oxaliplatin may be less appropriate in patients with pre-existing peripheral neuropathy (e.g., diabetics).

For patients with bulky symptomatic disease or where downstaging to potentially curative metastatectomy may be possible, combination first-line chemotherapy is usually considered in order to maximize objective tumor shrinkage. However, for patients with low-volume asymptomatic disease where there is no prospect of downstaging, first-line single-agent fluoropyrimidine may be considered, particularly if minimizing toxicity is desirable (e.g., elderly, comorbidity). If so, combination therapy may be added in the event of disease progression.

Although evidence relating to the optimal chemotherapy schedule for colorectal cancer from randomized controlled trials is not available, the accumulated data suggest that exposure to all three classes of drug (fluoropyrimidine, oxaliplatin, irinotecan) at some point in the course of the disease will optimize overall survival, with an improvement from 9 months with 5-FU to almost 2 years when all agents are used [86,87].

The duration of chemotherapy treatment is an area of ongoing research. Essentially there are two approaches. The first employs treatment until disease progression or intolerance. With combination chemotherapy in particular, cumulative toxicity (especially fatigue and oxaliplatin-related neurotoxicity) may frequently limit treatment duration. In order to address this problem the concept of a chemotherapy "holiday" may be employed, in which chemotherapy is administered for a fixed period (e.g., 3–6 months) followed by a planned break from treatment. When the tumor later progresses, the same regimen may then be reinstituted.

Inhibitors of EGF and VEGF in CRC

As with HCC, angiogenesis is key to CRC progression. Bevacizumab is a recombinant humanized monoclonal antibody that binds vascular endothelial growth factor, preventing its interaction with VEGF receptors. In patients with metastatic CRC, bevacizumab significantly prolongs survival when added to 5-FU, or to irinotecan-or oxaliplatin-based regimens [88,89]. Whilst the mechanism of action of bevacizumab is postulated to be anti-angiogenic, laboratory studies suggest it may increase blood flow through alterations in intratumoral interstitial pressure, thereby improving chemotherapy delivery to the tumor [90]. Combination chemotherapy with bevacizumab now represents a standard first-line treatment for metastatic CRC.

Aberrant epidermal growth-factor receptor (EGFR) signaling is implicated in 85% of CRC. In preclinical studies, cetuximab, an antibody against EGFR (Fig. 1.2), can reverse resistance to irinotecan, and a randomized phase II trial reported a response rate of 23% to the combination of cetuximab and irinotecan compared to 11% for cetuximab alone in patients with irinotecan-refractory disease [91]. More recently, the addition of cetuximab to first-line irinotecan-based therapy failed to significantly prolong overall survival. These data may be confounded by crossover. Indeed, there was a statistically significant increase in progression-free survival in the group receiving cetuximab [92]. The increasing complexity and expense of combination therapies necessitates the incorporation of translational research end points into clinical trials in order to guide treatment selection. This is exemplified by recent studies suggesting that, rather than the EGFR status of a tumor, the presence of wild-type Ras can predict responsiveness to cetuximab [93].

Downstaging of liver metastases

Since combination chemotherapy now consistently achieves objective responses in up to 50% of cases, the possibility of rendering initially unresectable disease resectable arises, and there are now several series in which this has been achieved in approximately 15% of cases, with 5-year survival similar to that of patients not requiring downstaging chemotherapy [94]. Several issues remain to be addressed. Both oxaliplatin- and irinotecan-based combinations can induce hepatic toxicity. Oxaliplatin can cause fatty liver and steatohepatitis, particularly in relation to pre-existing fatty liver and to duration of chemotherapy exposure. However, a recent randomized study investigating the role of neoadjuvant oxaliplatin-based chemotherapy prior to liver resection indicated that chemotherapy for 3 months before surgery was not associated with any significant increase in surgical morbidity or mortality [95]. Criteria for just which tumors are resectable are still evolving. The role of hepatic-artery infusion of cytotoxic agents for downstaging and systemic administration prior to resection of tumors for which there is no requirement for downstaging (i.e., in the neoadjuvant setting, with a view to limiting subsequent recurrence and extrahepatic disease) are both areas of ongoing research [95,96]. The integration of biological agents such as bevacizumab and cetuximab is also being investigated. Since the addition of these agents to conventional chemotherapy increases objective response rates, they may further increase the proportion of patients downstaged to resectability. However, this raises additional concerns regarding toxicity. In particular, since VEGF is known to play a critical role in wound healing and liver regeneration, bevacizumab should be used with caution in a preoperative setting, allowing sufficient time for its elimination before elective surgery.

Overall, the use of systemic therapies preoperatively requires balancing increased margin-negative resection, easier resections (e.g., segmentectomy rather than hemi-hepatectomy), and reduced recurrence through eradication of micrometastases against the risks of delaying surgery in non-responders and the adverse effects of chemotherapy on the liver.

Conclusions

Both HCC and CRC pose significant health burdens worldwide. Surgery remains the mainstay of treatment, offering the best prospect of long-term survival in both settings. Nevertheless, management can now be considered truly multidisciplinary. Identification of high-risk groups and advances in diagnostic radiology provide scope for earlier diagnosis and treatment. The interventional radiologist contributes local ablative techniques and regional chemotherapy delivery/embolization. In recent years there has been significant progress in systemic therapy for colorectal cancer. The introduction of more effective chemotherapy and newer biological agents has resulted in significant improvement in adjuvant therapy after primary surgery for colorectal cancer, reducing the risk of recurrence, better palliation for advanced disease, and, with higher objective response rates, the scope to downstage liver metastases and thereby expand the number of patients eligible for potentially curative interventions.

Identification of the major risk factors for HCC (chronic liver disease, chronic HBV and/or HCV infection, and aflatoxin exposure) has laid the foundation for screening and prevention.

Significant progress is being made in the prevention of hepatitis-B-related hepatocellular carcinoma (HCC), but hepatitis-C-related HCC is increasing in the West and therapeutic advances in established disease have been modest. Although transplantation, resection, and ablative therapies are effective in patients with small tumors they are only applicable to a minority of patients. Chemoembolization may offer useful palliation in a small subset of patients with excellent liver function and minimal symptoms.

Sorafenib is the first active systemic agent able to prolong survival for patients with advanced HCC, and this heralds an era of other novel agents and combinations to build on this breakthrough. The advent of active systemic therapies for HCC now opens up the possibility of their use as an adjuvant to surgery and other locoregional therapies, with the aim of decreasing recurrence/progression and as a bridge to liver transplant, where prevention of disease progression may be a valuable outcome.

REFERENCES

1. Parkin DM, Bray F, Ferlay J, Pisani P. Global cancer statistics, 2002. *CA Cancer J Clin* 2005; **55**: 74–108.
2. El-Serag HB. Epidemiology of hepatocellular carcinoma. *Clin Liver Dis* 2001; **5**: 87–107.
3. El-Serag HB, Mason AC. Rising incidence of hepatocellular carcinoma in the United States. *N Engl J Med* 1999; **340**: 745–50.
4. Johnson PJ. Risk factors for hepatocellular carcinoma. *ASCO 42nd Annual Meeting Educational Book* 2006, 234–7.
5. Chang MH, Chen CJ, Lai MS, *et al.* Universal hepatitis B vaccination in Taiwan and the incidence of hepatocellular carcinoma in children. Taiwan Childhood Hepatoma Study Group. *N Engl J Med* 1997; **336**: 1855–9.
6. Chan HL, Tse CH, Mo F, *et al.* High viral load and hepatitis B virus subgenotype ce are associated with increased risk of hepatocellular carcinoma. *J Clin Oncol* 2008; **26**: 177–82.
7. Liaw YF, Sung JJ, Chow WC, *et al.* Lamivudine for patients with chronic hepatitis B and advanced liver disease. *N Engl J Med* 2004; **351**: 1521–31.

8. Sun CA, Wu DM, Lin CC, *et al.* Incidence and cofactors of hepatitis C virus-related hepatocellular carcinoma: a prospective study of 12,008 men in Taiwan. *Am J Epidemiol* 2003; **157**: 674–82.

9. Yu ML, Lin SM, Chuang WL, *et al.* A sustained virological response to interferon or interferon/ribavirin reduces hepatocellular carcinoma and improves survival in chronic hepatitis C: a nationwide, multicentre study in Taiwan. *Antivir Ther* 2006; **11**: 985–94.

10. Bruno S, Crosignani A, Maisonneuve P, *et al.* Hepatitis C virus genotype 1B as a major risk factor associated with hepatocellular carcinoma in patients with cirrhosis: a seventeen-year prospective cohort study. *Hepatology* 2007; **46**: 1350–6.

11. Johnson PJ, Williams R. Cirrhosis and the aetiology of hepatocellular carcinoma. *J Hepatol* 1987; **4**: 140–7.

12. Kensler TW, Egner PA, Wang JB, *et al.* Chemoprevention of hepatocellular carcinoma in aflatoxin endemic areas. *Gastroenterology* 2004; **127** (5 Suppl 1): S310–18.

13. Turner PC, Sylla A, Gong YY, *et al.* Reduction in exposure to carcinogenic aflatoxins by postharvest intervention measures in West Africa: a community-based intervention study. *Lancet* 2005; **365**: 1950–6.

14. Lai EC, Lau WY. Spontaneous rupture of hepatocellular carcinoma: a systematic review. *Arch Surg* 2006; **141**: 191–8.

15. McFadzean AJ, Todd D, Tso SC. Erythrocytosis associated with hepatocellular carcinoma. *Blood* 1967; **29**: 808–11.

16. Bruix J, Sherman M, Llovet JM, *et al.* EASL panel of experts on HCC. Clinical management of hepatocellular carcinoma: conclusions of the Barcelona-2000 EASL conference. *J Hepatol* 2001; **35**: 421–30.

17. Bhattacharjya S, Bhattacharjya T, Quaglia A, *et al.* Liver transplantation in cirrhotic patients with small hepatocellular carcinoma: an analysis of pre-operative imaging, explant histology and prognostic histologic indicators. *Dig Surg* 2004; **21**: 152–9.

18. Johnson PJ. The role of serum alpha-fetoprotein estimation in the diagnosis and management of hepatocellular carcinoma. *Clin Liver Dis* 2001; **5**: 145–59.

19. Okuda K. Natural history of hepatocellular carcinoma including fibrolamellar and hepato-cholangiocarcinoma variants. *J Gastroenterol Hepatol* 2002; **17**: 401–5.

20. Chen JG, Parkin DM, Chen QG, *et al.* Screening for liver cancer: results of a randomised controlled trial in Qidong, China. *J Med Screen* 2003; **10**: 204–9.

21. Bruix J, Sherman M. Practice Guidelines Committee, American Association for the Study of Liver Diseases. Management of hepatocellular carcinoma. *Hepatology* 2005; **42**: 1208–36.

22. Sherman M. Hepatocellular carcinoma: epidemiology, risk factors, and screening. *Semin Liver Dis* 2005; **25**: 143–54.

23. Thompson Coon J, Rogers G, Hewson P, *et al.* Surveillance of cirrhosis for hepatocellular carcinoma: systematic review and economic analysis. *Health Technol Assess* 2007; **11**: 1–206.

24. Palmer DH, Johnson PJ. Hepatocellular carcinoma. In: Gospodarowicz MK, O'Sullivan B, Sobin LH, eds. *Prognostic Factors in Cancer*, 3rd edn. Hoboken, NJ: Wiley, 2006, 143–6.

25. Ebara M, Ohto M, Shinagawa T, *et al.* Natural history of minute hepatocellular carcinoma smaller than three centimeters complicating cirrhosis: a study in 22 patients. *Gastroenterology* 1986; **90**: 289–98.

26. Wayne JD, Lauwers GY, Ikai I, *et al.* Preoperative predictors of survival after resection of small hepatocellular carcinomas. *Ann Surg* 2002; **235**: 722–30.

27. Poon RT, Ng IO, Fan ST, *et al.* Clinicopathologic features of long-term survivors and disease-free survivors after resection of hepatocellular carcinoma: a study of a prospective cohort. *J Clin Oncol* 2001; **19**: 3037–44.

28. Farmer DG, Rosove MH, Shaket A, *et al.* Current treatment modalities for hepatocellular carcinoma. *Ann Surg* 1994; **219**: 236–47.

29. Vauthey JN, Klimstra D, Franceschi D, *et al.* Factors affecting long-term outcome after hepatic resection for hepatocellular carcinoma. *Am J Surg* 1995; **169**: 28–34.

30. Mazzaferro V, Regalia E, Doci R, *et al.* Liver transplantation for the treatment of small hepatocellular carcinomas in patients with cirrhosis. *N Engl J Med* 1996; **334**: 693–9.

31. Yao FY, Ferrell L, Bass NM, *et al.* Liver transplantation for hepatocellular carcinoma: expansion of the tumor size limits does not adversely impact survival. *Hepatology* 2001; **33**: 1394–403.

32. Yao FY, Bass NM, Nikolai B, *et al.* A follow-up analysis of the pattern and predictors of dropout from the waiting list for liver transplantation in patients with hepatocellular carcinoma: implications for the current organ allocation policy. *Liver Transpl* 2003; **9**: 684–92.

33. United Network for Organ Sharing. www.unos.org.

34. Gondolesi GE, Roayaie S, Munoz L, *et al.* Adult living donor liver transplantation for patients with hepatocellular carcinoma: extending UNOS priority criteria. *Ann Surg* 2004; **239**: 42–9.

35. Palmer DH, Johnson PJ. Pre-operative locoregional therapy and liver transplantation for hepatocellular carcinoma (HCC): time for a randomised controlled trial. *Am J Transplant* 2005; **5**: 641–2.

36. Livraghi T, Giorgio A, Marin G, *et al.* Hepatocellular carcinoma and cirrhosis in 746 patients: long-term results of percutaneous ethanol injection. *Radiology* 1995; **197**: 101–8.

37. Shiina S, Teratani T, Obi S, *et al.* A randomized controlled trial of radiofrequency ablation with ethanol injection for small hepatocellular carcinoma. *Gastroenterology*, 2005; **129**: 122–30.

38. Lencioni R, Cioni C, Crocetti L, *et al.* Early-stage hepatocellular carcinoma in patients with cirrhosis: long-term results of percutaneous image-guided radiofrequency ablation. *Radiology* 2005; **234**: 961–7.

39. Livraghi T, Goldberg SN, Lazzaroni S, *et al.* Small hepatocellular carcinoma: treatment with radio-frequency ablation versus ethanol injection. *Radiology* 1999; **210**: 655–61.

40. Chen HS, Gross JF. Intra-arterial infusion of anticancer drugs: theoretic aspects of drug delivery and review of responses. *Cancer Treat Rep* 1980; **64**: 31–40.

41. Yumoto Y, Jinno K, Tokuyama K, *et al.* Hepatocellular carcinoma detected by iodized oil. *Radiology* 1985; **154**: 19–24.

42. Brown DB, Geschwind JF, Soulen MC, *et al.* Society of Interventional Radiology position statement on chemoembolization for hepatic malignancies. *J Vasc Intervent Radiol* 2006; **17**: 217–23.

43. Lo CM, Ngan H, Tso WK, *et al.* Randomized controlled trial of transarterial lipiodol chemoembolization for unresectable hepatocellular carcinoma. *Hepatology* 2002; **35**: 1164–71.
44. Llovet JM, Real MI, Montana X, *et al.* Barcelona Clinic Liver Cancer Group. Arterial embolisation or chemoembolisation versus symptomatic treatment in patients with unresectable hepatocellular carcinoma: a randomized controlled trial. *Lancet* 2002; **359**: 1734–9.
45. Bruix J, Sala M, Llovet JM. Chemoembolization for hepatocellular carcinoma. *Gastroenterology* 2004; **127**: S179–88.
46. Simonetti RG, Leberati A, Angiolini C, *et al.* Treatment of hepatocellular carcinoma: a systematic review of randomized controlled trials. *Ann Oncol* 1997; **8**: 117–36.
47. Palmer DH, Hussain SA, Johnson PJ. Systemic therapies for hepatocellular carcinoma. *Expert Opin Investig Drugs* 2004; **3**: 1555–68.
48. Gish RG, Porta C, Lazar L, *et al.* Phase III randomized controlled trial comparing the survival of patients with unresectable hepatocellular carcinoma treated with nolatrexed or doxorubicin. *J Clin Oncol* 2007; **25**: 3069–75.
49. Yeo W, Mok TS, Zee B, *et al.* A randomized phase III study of doxorubicin versus cisplatin/interferon alpha-2b/doxorubicin/fluorouracil (PIAF) combination chemotherapy for unresectable hepatocellular carcinoma. *J Nat Cancer Inst* 2005; **97**: 1532–8.
50. Barbare JC, Bouche O, Bonnetain F, *et al.* Randomized controlled trial of tamoxifen in advanced hepatocellular carcinoma. *J Clin Oncol* 2005; **23**: 4338–46.
51. CLIP Group (Cancer of the Liver Italian Programme). Tamoxifen in treatment of hepatocellular carcinoma: a randomised controlled trial. *Lancet* 1998; **352**: 17–20.
52. Reynaert H, Rombouts K, Vandermonde A, *et al.* Expression of somatostatin receptors in normal and cirrhotic human liver and in hepatocellular carcinoma. *Gut* 2004; **53**: 1180–9.
53. Blaker M, Schmitz M, Gocht A, *et al.* Differential expression of somatostatin receptor subtypes in hepatocellular carcinomas. *J Hepatol* 2004; **41**: 112–18.
54. Kouroumalis E, Skordilis P, Thermos K, *et al.* Treatment of hepatocellular carcinoma with octreotide: a randomised controlled study. *Gut* 1998; **42**: 442–7.
55. Yuen MF, Poon RT, Lai CL, *et al.* A randomized placebo-controlled study of long-acting octreotide for the treatment of advanced hepatocellular carcinoma. *Hepatology* 2002; **36**: 687–91.
56. Becker G, Allgaier HP, Olschewski M, *et al.* Long-acting octreotide versus placebo for treatment of advanced HCC: a randomized controlled double-blind study. *Hepatology* 2007; **45**: 9–15.
57. Yamaguchi R, Yano H, Iemura A, *et al.* Expression of vascular endothelial growth factor in human hepatocellular carcinoma. *Hepatology* 1998; **28**: 68–77.
58. Chao Y, Li CP, Chau GY, *et al.* Prognostic significance of vascular endothelial growth factor, basic fibroblast growth factor, and angiogenin in patients with resectable hepatocellular carcinoma after surgery. *Ann Surg Oncol* 2003; **10**: 355–62.
59. Ito Y, Sasaki Y, Horimoto M, *et al.* Activation of mitogen-activated protein kinases/extracellular signal-regulated kinases in human hepatocellular carcinoma. *Hepatology* 1998; **27**: 951–8.

60. Abou-Alfa GK, Schwartz L, Ricci S, *et al.* Phase II study of sorafenib in patients with advanced hepatocellular carcinoma. *J Clin Oncol* 2006; **24**: 4293–300.

61. Llovet J, Ricci S, Mazzaferro V, *et al.* SHARP Investigators Study Group. Sorafenib improves survival in advanced hepatocellular carcinoma (HCC): results of a phase III randomized placebo-controlled trial (SHARP trial). *J Clin Oncol* 2007; **25**. ASCO Annual Meeting Proceedings LBA1.

62. Zhu AX, Sahani DV, di Tomaso E, *et al.* A phase II study of sunitinib in patients with advanced hepatocellular carcinoma. *J Clin Oncol* 2007; **25**: 4637.

63. Schwartz J, Schwartz M, Lehrer D, *et al.* Bevacizumab in hepatocellular carcinoma (HCC) in patients without metastases and without portal vein invasion. *J Clin Oncol* 2005; **23**: 4122.

64. Abbruzzese JL, Thomas MB. Opportunities for targeted therapies in hepatocellular carcinoma. *J Clin Oncol* 2005; **23**: 8093–108.

65. Philip PA, Mahoney MR, Allmer C, *et al.* Phase II study of erlotinib (OSI-774) in patients with advanced hepatocellular cancer. *J Clin Oncol* 2005; **23**: 6657–63.

66. Thomas MB, Dutta D, Brown T, *et al.* A phase II open-label study of OSI-774 (NSC 718781) in unresectable hepatocellular carcinoma. *Proc Am Soc Clin Oncol* 2005; **23**: 4083a.

67. Thomas MB, Chadha R, Iwasaki M, *et al.* The combination of bevacizumab (B) and erlotinib (E) shows significant biological activity in patients with advanced hepatocellular carcinoma (HCC). *J Clin Oncol* 2007; **25**: 4567.

68. Abou-Alfa G, Johnson P, Knox J, *et al.* Preliminary results from a phase II, randomized, double-blind study of sorafenib plus doxorubicin versus placebo plus doxorubicin in patients with advanced hepatocellular carcinoma. *Eur J Cancer* 2007; **5** (Suppl): Abst 3500.

69. Hawkins MA, Dawson LA. Radiation therapy for hepatocellular carcinoma: from palliation to cure. *Cancer* 2006; **106**: 1653–63.

70. Robertson JM, Lawrence TS, Dworzanin LM, *et al.* Treatment of primary hepatobiliary cancers with conformal radiation therapy and regional chemotherapy. *J Clin Oncol* 1993; **1**: 1286–93.

71. Raoul JI, Bretagne JF, Caucanas JP, *et al.* Internal radiation therapy for hepatocellular carcinoma: results of a French multicenter phase II trial of transarterial injection of iodine 131-labeled lipiodol. *Cancer* 1992; **69**: 346–52.

72. Lau WY, Ho S, Leung TW, *et al.* Selective internal radiation therapy for nonresectable hepatocellular carcinoma with intraarterial infusion of ^{90}yttrium microspheres. *Int J Radiat Oncol Biol Phys* 1998; **40**: 583–92.

73. Bhattacharjya S, Bhattacharjya T, Baber S, *et al.* Prospective study of contrast-enhanced computed tomography, computed tomography during arterioportography, and magnetic resonance imaging for staging colorectal liver metastases for liver resection. *Br J Surg* 2004; **91**: 1361–9.

74. Wagner JS, Adson MA, Van Heerden JA, *et al.* The natural history of hepatic metastases from colorectal cancer: a comparison with resective treatment. *Ann Surg* 1984; **199**: 502–8.

75. Simmonds PC, Primrose JN, Colquitt JL, *et al.* Surgical resection of hepatic metastases from colorectal cancer: a systematic review of published studies. *Br J Cancer* 2006; **94**: 982–99.

76. Oshowo A, Gillams A, Harrison E, *et al.* Comparison of resection and radiofrequency ablation for treatment of solitary colorectal liver metastases. *Br J Surg* 2003; **90**: 1240–3.

77. The Meta-Analysis Group in Cancer. Modulation of fluorouracil by leucovorin in patients with advanced colorectal cancer: an updated meta-analysis. *J Clin Oncol* 2004; **22**: 3766–75.

78. Van Cutsem E, Twelves C, Cassidy J, *et al.* Colorectal Cancer Study Group. Oral capecitabine compared with intravenous fluorouracil plus leucovorin in patients with metastatic colorectal cancer: results of a large phase III study. *J Clin Oncol* 2001; **19**: 4097–106.

79. Cunningham D, Pyrhonen S, James RD, *et al.* Randomised trial of irinotecan plus supportive care versus supportive care alone after fluorouracil failure for patients with metastatic colorectal cancer. *Lancet* 1998; **352**: 1413–8.

80. Saltz LB, Cox JV, Blanke C, *et al.* Irinotecan plus fluorouracil and leucovorin for metastatic colorectal cancer. Irinotecan Study Group. *N Engl J Med* 2000; **343**: 905–14.

81. Douillard JY, Cunningham D, Roth AD, *et al.* Irinotecan combined with fluorouracil compared with fluorouracil alone as first-line treatment for metastatic colorectal cancer: a multicentre randomised trial. *Lancet* 2000; **355**: 1041–7.

82. Rothenberg ML, Meropol NJ, Poplin EA, *et al.* Mortality associated with irinotecan plus bolus fluorouracil/leucovorin: summary findings of an independent panel. *J Clin Oncol* 2002; **20**: 1145–6.

83. de Gramont A, Vignoud J, Tournigand C, *et al.* Oxaliplatin with high-dose leucovorin and 5-fluorouracil 48-hour continuous infusion in pretreated metastatic colorectal cancer. *Eur J Cancer* 1997; **33**: 214–19.

84. de Gramont A, Figer A, Seymour M, *et al.* Leucovorin and fluorouracil with or without oxaliplatin as first-line treatment in advanced colorectal cancer. *J Clin Oncol* 2000; **18**: 2938–47.

85. Goldberg RM, Sargent DJ, Morton RF, *et al.* A randomized controlled trial of fluorouracil plus leucovorin, irinotecan, and oxaliplatin combinations in patients with previously untreated metastatic colorectal cancer. *J Clin Oncol* 2004; **22**: 23–30.

86. Tournigand C, Andre T, Achille E, *et al.* FOLFIRI followed by FOLFOX6 or the reverse sequence in advanced colorectal cancer: a randomized GERCOR study. *J Clin Oncol* 2004; **22**: 229–37.

87. Kelly H, Goldberg RM. Systemic therapy for metastatic colorectal cancer: current options, current evidence. *J Clin Oncol* 2005; **23**: 4553–60.

88. Hurwitz HI, Fehrenbacher L, Novotny W, *et al.* Bevacizumab in combination with fluorouracil and leucovorin: an active regimen for first-line metastatic colorectal cancer. *J Clin Oncol* 2005; **23**: 3502–8.

89. Kabbinavar FF, Schulz J, McCleod M, *et al.* Addition of bevacizumab to bolus fluorouracil and leucovorin in first-line metastatic colorectal cancer: results of a randomized phase II trial. *J Clin Oncol* 2005; **23**: 3697–705.

90. Jain RK. Normalization of tumor vasculature: an emerging concept in antiangiogenic therapy. *Science* 2005; **307**: 58–62.

91. Cunningham D, Humblet Y, Siena S, *et al.* Cetuximab monotherapy and cetuximab plus irinotecan in irinotecan-refractory metastatic colorectal cancer. *N Engl J Med* 2004; **351**: 337–45.

92. Van Cutsem E, Nowacki M, Lang I, *et al.* Randomized phase III study of irinotecan and 5-FU/FA with or without cetuximab in the first-line treatment of patients with metastatic colorectal cancer (mCRC): the CRYSTAL trial. *J Clin Oncol* 2007; **25** (18S): 4000.

93. De Roock W, Piessevaux H, De Schutter J, *et al.* KRAS wild-type state predicts survival and is associated to early radiological response in metastatic colorectal cancer treated with cetuximab. *Ann Oncol* 2008; **19**: 508–15.

94. Leonard GD, Brenner B, Kemeny NE. Neoadjuvant chemotherapy before liver resection for patients with unresectable liver metastases from colorectal carcinoma. *J Clin Oncol* 2005; **23**: 2038–48.

95. Nordlinger N, Sorbye H, Collette L, *et al.* Final results of the EORTC Intergroup randomized phase III study 40983 [EPOC] evaluating the benefit of peri-operative FOLFOX4 chemotherapy for patients with potentially resectable colorectal cancer liver metastases. *J Clin Oncol* 2007; **25** (18S): LBA5.

96. Kemeny NE, Niedzwiecki D, Hollis DR, *et al.* Hepatic arterial infusion versus systemic therapy for hepatic metastases from colorectal cancer: a randomized trial of efficacy, quality of life, and molecular markers (CALGB 9481). *J Clin Oncol* 2006; **24**: 1395–403.

2

Pathology of hepatocellular carcinoma and hepatic metastases

Masamichi Kojiro

Introduction

Previously, hepatocellular carcinoma (HCC) was a major problem only in Asian and African countries, but it has become a common problem for gastroentero- logists, radiologists, and pathologists in Western countries as well. Until 30 years ago most HCCs were detected at an advanced stage, and the survival time after diagnosis was no longer than 1 year. Remarkable advances in clinical diagnostic approaches, in particular the development of various diagnostic imaging techniques and the establishment of a follow-up system for high-risk populations, have made it possible to detect small HCCs at an early stage. The characteristic clinicopathologic features of early-stage HCC, which are very different than those of classical advanced-stage HCC, have now been well documented in humans, and much has been discovered about the process of hepatocarcinogenesis and the morphological evolution from early to advanced HCC. The most characteristic pathological feature of small early-stage HCCs, up to around 2.0 cm in diameter, is that many of them are well differentiated. Such well-differentiated small HCCs are not yet encapsu- lated and contain portal tracts inside the nodule, meaning that they receive portal blood supply as well. Well-differentiated HCCs at the early stage show dediffer- entiation along with an increase in tumor size, and many HCCs larger than 3 cm become moderately differentiated and show the clinicopathologic features of classical HCC.

Pathology of hepatocellular carcinoma

The establishment of a follow-up system for patients at high risk for the develop- ment of hepatocellular carcinoma and advances in diagnostic imaging techniques in

Interventional Radiological Treatment of Liver Tumors, ed. Andy Adam and Peter R. Mueller.
Published by Cambridge University Press. © Cambridge University Press 2009.

recent years have led to the detection of an increasing number of small nodular lesions of the liver. While some of these nodules represent well-differentiated HCC at an early stage, in other cases the material obtained is histologically insufficient or equivocal for a diagnosis of HCC. These small nodular lesions have started to attract the attention of both histopathologists and clinicians. A substantial volume of clinical and pathological information relating to early-stage HCC and equivocal nodular lesions has been obtained during the last two decades [1–22]. However, despite substantial progress, many HCCs are still detected at an advanced stage, particularly in areas where effective follow-up systems for high-risk populations have not been established.

Premalignant lesions of HCC

With an increasing number of HCCs treated by surgical resection and liver transplantation, equivocal small nodules have become a matter of interest for both pathologists and physicians. In 1995, the International Working Party Classification [23] proposed the term "dysplastic nodule" for equivocal nodular lesions in a cirrhotic liver, and this is now widely used.

Dysplastic nodules

A dysplastic nodule (DN) is defined grossly as a hepatic nodule that is distinct from surrounding regenerative nodules in terms of size, color, and texture. Histologically, DNs show varying degrees of increased cell density, with a distinct trabecular arrangement, and retain portal tracts within them. They are subclassified into low-grade and high-grade DNs according to the degree of cellular and structural atypia.

Low-grade DNs are well defined but not encapsulated, approximately 1.0 cm in diameter and slightly more yellow than their surroundings. The hepatocytes are minimally abnormal, and apparently normal portal tracts are present in the nodules. The nuclear/cytoplasmic (N/C) ratio is slightly increased, and cell density is no more than twice that of surrounding liver [21] (Fig. 2.1a). Marked iron deposition is sometimes observed [24]. DNs have been said to consist of monoclonal cell expansion with genetic alterations [25–28]. Morphologic differentiation from well-differentiated HCC is not difficult in most cases.

High-grade DNs are usually vaguely nodular, and are difficult to differentiate from early-stage well-differentiated HCC on gross examination. Histologically, high-grade DNs are characterized by cell density more than twice as high as that

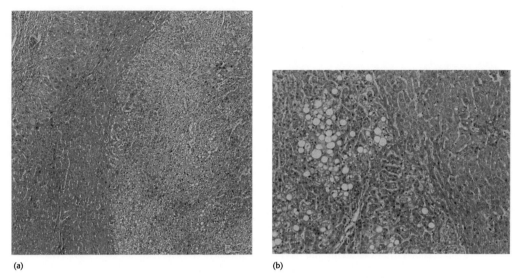

(a)   (b)

Figure 2.1 Dysplastic nodule. (a) Low-grade dysplastic nodule: a nodule (right half) shows mildly increased cell density and clearer trabecular arrangement in parts. (b) High-grade dysplastic nodule: a nodule (left half) shows markedly increased cell density with an irregular trabecular arrangement and fatty change. *See color plate section.*

of the surrounding liver, an irregular thin-trabecular pattern, and occasional unpaired arteries. It is often difficult to distinguish high-grade DN from well-differentiated HCC (Fig. 2.1b). In high-grade DN, sinusoidal endothelial cells are immunohistochemically positive to CD34 only in parts of the lesion (incomplete sinusoidal capillarization) [29,30]. On contrast-enhanced CT or MRI, high-grade DNs are hypovascular. Occasionally, high-grade DNs contain foci of well-differentiated HCC, the presence of which strongly suggests that DN is a precancerous lesion [31,32]. In addition, follow-up studies have revealed that a considerable number of high-grade DNs evolve into classical HCCs within a few years [5,6].

Early-stage well-differentiated HCC

Morphologic characteristics of small HCC of early stage
Small HCCs, up to around 2 cm in diameter, are classified into two major types; the distinctly nodular type and the vaguely nodular type [12,33] (Fig. 2.2). Histologically, most of the distinctly nodular HCCs are moderately differentiated, whereas the majority of the vaguely nodular type are very well differentiated. It is

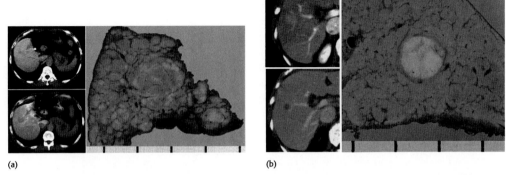

(a)   (b)

Figure 2.2 Small HCC. (a) Vaguely nodular type: a tumor measuring 1.7 × 1.5 cm is vaguely nodular and retained portal tracts are recognizable; it is hypovascular on contrast CT. (b) Distinctly nodular type: a tumor of 1.2 cm in diameter is distinctly nodular and well encapsulated. On contrast CT, a tumor shows hypervascularity and "wash-out" as seen in classical HCC. *See color plate section.*

important to understand the clinicopathological differences between these two types, because they are remarkably different not only morphologically but also biologically.

Small HCCs of the vaguely nodular type are visualized as a distinct hypoechoic or hyperechoic nodular lesion on ultrasonography, and they appear hypovascular on contrast-enhanced CT (Fig. 2.2a). Most of these lesions are indistinct in the resected specimen, and the indistinctness of the tumor is caused by a replacing growth at the tumor boundary, as if the tumor cells are replacing the surrounding liver cell cords. The vaguely nodular small HCC consists of well-differentiated HCC tissues, and variable numbers of portal tracts are retained within the tumor (Fig. 2.3). However, the number of intratumoral portal tracts is less than one-third of those of the surrounding liver tissue [34], and many of the retained portal tracts are deformed due to varying degrees of tumor-cell invasion, which is designated as "stromal invasion." This stromal invasion is regarded as the most helpful clue to distinguishing small well-differentiated HCC from high-grade DN [35,36] (Fig. 2.4).

Most vaguely nodular small HCCs receive both portal blood and arterial blood from the arterial tumor vessels (unpaired arteries), hepatic arteries, and portal veins in the intratumoral portal tracts [34]. However, the portal blood supply is signifi-cantly reduced compared to that in the surrounding liver tissue, because there are fewer portal tracts than in the surrounding tissue [34,37]. The hypovascularity of the vaguely nodular type is explained by the insufficient development of unpaired

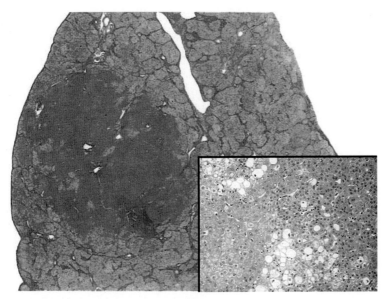

Figure 2.3 Histological findings of vaguely nodular small HCC. The tumor consists of uniformly distributed well-differentiated HCC tissue with retained portal tracts, and shows a replacing growth at the tumor boundary without forming a capsule (inset). *See color plate section.*

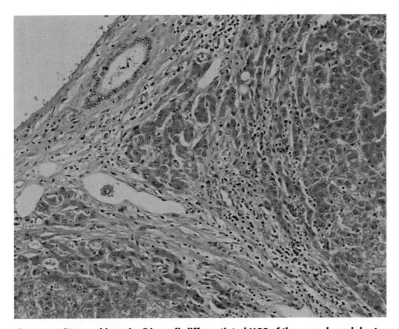

Figure 2.4 "Stromal invasion" in well-differentiated HCC of the vaguely nodular type. This tumor-cell infiltration into the portal tract within the tumor is a helpful morphologic clue in distinguishing well-differentiated HCC from high-grade DN. *See color plate section.*

arteries, the lack of fibrous capsule, and incomplete capillarization of sinusoid-like blood spaces. The average number of unpaired arteries per square millimetre in early-stage HCC is less than half that of advanced HCC, and capillarization of the sinusoids is only focally observed [28,29].

Small HCC is often hyperechoic because it contains diffuse fatty change. Diffuse fatty change occupying more than about a third of the area of the mass is most frequent (42.4%) in tumors measuring 1.1–1.5 cm in diameter, especially in well-differentiated masses of the vaguely nodular type, whereas it is found in only 18.8% of tumors smaller than 1 cm and in 15.5% of tumors larger than 3 cm in diameter. It may be caused by a temporal ischemia due to an insufficient arterial blood supply [19].

Small HCCs of the distinctly nodular type show expansive growth, and many are encapsulated (Fig. 2.2b). Histologically, most are moderately differentiated and there are no retained portal tracts. Unpaired arteries and capillarization of the sinusoid-like blood spaces are well developed, and the tumors are visualized as hypervascular nodules on contrast-enhanced imaging [15]. Therefore, the distinctly nodular small HCC is no different from classical HCC, despite its small size.

Evolution of HCC from early to advanced stage

Morphologic studies of resected HCCs of various sizes and biopsy material from small HCCs at an early stage of development have shown that small well-differentiated HCC demonstrates gradual dedifferentiation [17,21]. HCC often has histological variations in a single tumor nodule. Although vaguely nodular HCCs smaller than 1.5 cm in diameter consist uniformly of well-differentiated cancerous tissue, about 40% of HCC nodules 1.5–3cm in diameter are composed of tumor tissue of at least two different histological grades, mostly well-differentiated and moderately differentiated. Less differentiated tumor tissue is usually surrounded by well-differentiated tumor tissue. As the tumor increases in size, the area of well-differentiated tumor tissues diminishes and is eventually replaced by less differentiated tumor tissue [38].

"Nodule–in–nodule" appearance. When well-differentiated HCC nodules contain less differentiated tumor tissue expanding with a clear boundary, they often show a "nodule-in-nodule" appearance, which is the morphologic expression of dedifferentiation in well-differentiated HCC [33]. A "nodule-in-nodule" appearance is easily appreciated on diagnostic imaging. In particular, when

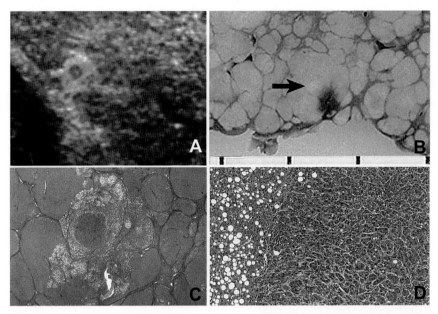

Figure 2.5 A "nodule-in-nodule" appearance in early-stage HCC. (a) On ultrasound, a tumor shows a hypoechoic subnodule within a hyperechoic tumor. (b) Grossly, a tumor measuring 1 cm in diameter contains a minute whitish nodule (arrow). (c, d) Histologically, an outer nodule consists of well-differentiated HCC with fatty change, and a subnodule consists of moderately differentiated HCC without fatty change. *See color plate section.*

well-differentiated HCC with fatty change contains less differentiated tissue without fatty change, it is visualized on ultrasound studies as a hyperechoic tumor containing a well-demarcated hypoechoic nodule (Fig. 2.5). A hypoechoic nodule inside a hyperechoic one gradually increases in size, and eventually the hyperechoic areas disappear.

Pathology of advanced HCC

Gross appearance

According to Eggel's classification there are three major types of classical HCC at an advanced stage: nodular, massive, and diffuse [39]. The commonest is the nodular type, which often has a fibrous capsule (Fig. 2.6a). It is often associated with various degrees of extranodular tumor growth and/or satellite nodules including intrahepatic metastases. Massive-type tumor usually occupies the entire right or left hepatic lobe (Fig. 2.6b). Large nodular tumors may also occupy an entire lobe,

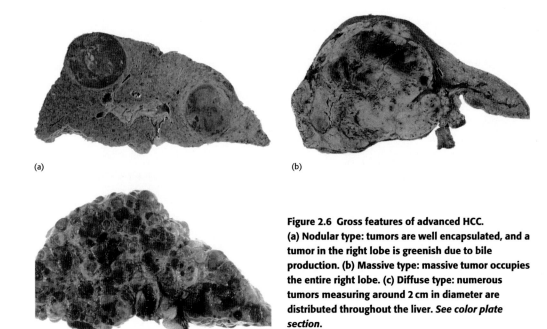

(a)

(b)

(c)

Figure 2.6 Gross features of advanced HCC.
(a) Nodular type: tumors are well encapsulated, and a tumor in the right lobe is greenish due to bile production. (b) Massive type: massive tumor occupies the entire right lobe. (c) Diffuse type: numerous tumors measuring around 2 cm in diameter are distributed throughout the liver. *See color plate section*.

mimicking a massive-type mass. Diffuse tumors are relatively infrequent, and replace the entire liver with diffusely distributed tumor nodules 1–2 cm in size (Fig. 2.6c). This type of HCC is occasionally misdiagnosed as liver cirrhosis on ultrasonographic examination.

Histological findings

Histologically, HCC is basically composed of tumor cells in a trabecular arrangement (tumor parenchyma) and sinusoid-like blood spaces (tumor stroma). The thickness of the trabeculae is correlated with tumor differentiation: thinner in well-differentiated HCC and thicker in less differentiated tumor. Some HCCs have tumor cells exhibiting biliary markers such as cytokeratin (CK) 7 and 19 positivity, which are suggestive of hepatic progenitor cell origin and are associated with a poor prognosis [40–43].

In **well-differentiated HCC**, tumor cells with little cellular atypia are arranged in a trabecular pattern 2–3 cells thick, with occasional pseudoglands (Fig. 2.7a). When

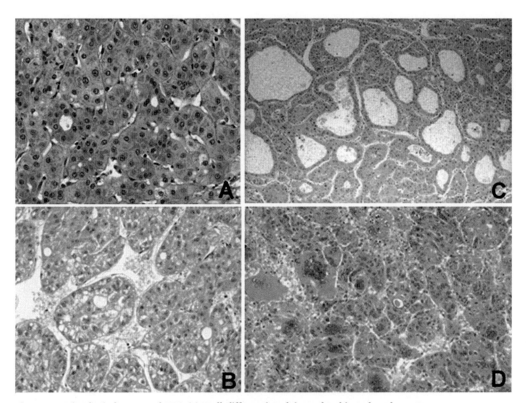

Figure 2.7 Histologic features of HCC. (a) Well-differentiated: irregular thin trabecular pattern with occasional pseudoglands is characteristic. (b) Moderately differentiated: tumor shows varying sized tumor-cell islands (trabeculae) as if they are floating in sinusoidal blood spaces. (c) Pseudoglandular type: varying sized pseudoglands containing protein-like fluid are frequently observed in moderately differentiated HCC, and HCC with a prominent pseudoglandular pattern is called pseudoglandular type. (d) Poorly differentiated: tumor consists of mononuclear and/or multinuclear bizarre giant cells with a vague trabecular or solid pattern, and it is also called giant-cell HCC.
See color plate section.

well-differentiated tumor tissue is present in advanced HCC, it is found only in the periphery of the tumor. Rarely, a large HCC consists solely of well-differentiated tumor tissue, and in such cases the differentiation from liver cell adenoma is problematic.

In **moderately differentiated HCC** the tumor shows cell islands (trabeculae) of varying sizes, apparently floating in sinusoidal blood spaces. This pattern is regarded as a classical form of HCC (Fig. 2.7b). Pseudoglands containing proteinaceous fluid or bile are frequently observed in moderately differentiated HCC. HCC which exhibits prominent pseudoglands is called HCC of *pseudoglandular type* (Fig. 2.7c).

Poorly differentiated HCCs exhibit either a solid growth pattern or a prominent pleomorphic pattern. Solid-pattern tumors contain cells with a high nuclear/cytoplasm ratio arranged in sheets, without trabeculae, accompanied by a small number of slit-like arteries. Pleomorphic-pattern HCC consists of mononuclear and/or multinuclear bizarre giant cells with a vague trabecular or solid pattern, and may also be classified as *giant-cell* HCC (Fig. 2.7d).

Variants of HCC

Fibrolamellar carcinoma (FLC) is a variant of HCC with characteristic clinico-pathological features. The incidence of FLC is geographically different, and it is rare in Asia. FLC is not associated with liver cirrhosis, and frequently occurs in adolescents or young adults, with a mean age of 23 years [44]. The prognosis is better than that of classical HCC. Grossly, the tumor is well demarcated but not encapsulated, and it is greyish white in colour. One of the characteristic findings is the frequent presence of a central fibrous scar with radiating fibrous bands dividing the tumor into lobules, thus mimicking focal nodular hyperplasia (Fig. 2.8a). Histologically, FLC consists of the tumor cells with abundant deeply eosinophilic cytoplasm and distinct nucleolus growing in sheets or small trabeculae, which are separated by fibrous collagen with a lamellar pattern and frequent hyalinization. A characteristic intracytoplasmic inclusion "pale body" that is immunohistochemically positive to antifibrinogen is frequently observed [45,46] (Fig. 2.8b).

Scirrhous HCC is characterized by diffuse fibrosis along sinusoidal blood spaces with varying degrees of atrophy of tumor trabeculae in the absence of a history of previous anti-cancer therapy (Fig. 2.9a). Scirrhous HCC is found in 4.6% of surgical cases [47]. On diagnostic imaging, scirrhous HCC is frequently misdiagnosed as cholangiocarcinoma, combined hepatocellular and cholangiocellular carcinoma, or metastatic carcinoma.

Sarcomatoid (sarcomatous) HCC is characterized by the proliferation of short spindle-shaped sarcomatous cells and/or bizarre giant cells, and it is found in 1.9% of resected HCCs [48] and 6.4% of autopsy cases [49–51] (Fig. 2.9b). When there are no transitional features between classical HCC tissue and sarcomatous tissue, it is sometimes difficult to differentiate from a true sarcoma.

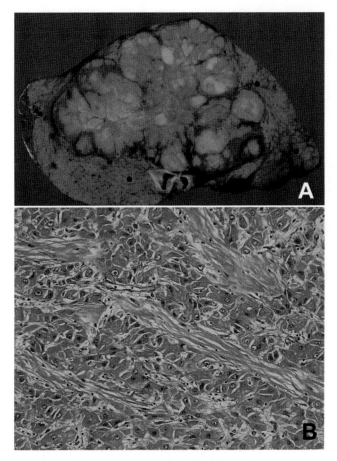

Figure 2.8 Fibrolamellar carcinoma. (a) Gross appearance: tumor shows a central fibrous scar with radiating fibrous bands dividing the tumor into lobules, mimicking focal nodular hyperplasia. (b) Histologically, the tumor cells have abundant and deeply eosinophilic cytoplasm with round nuclei having distinct nucleoli. The tumor grows in sheets or small trabeculae, which are separated by fibrous collagen with a characteristic lamellar pattern. *See color plate section.*

Angioarchitecture of advanced HCC

HCC typically receives arterial blood exclusively via arterial tumor vessels (unpaired arteries), whereas the branches of the portal vein stay along the tumor boundaries (capsule).

Arterial tumor vessels (unpaired arteries)

The arterial tumor vessels in HCC have a variable thickness of smooth muscle in the vessel wall and are also called "unpaired arteries." The development of arterial tumor vessels follows tumor growth (Fig. 2.10). The number of such vessels in small HCC of the vaguely nodular type is only one-third of that observed in classical HCC, but it is similar to that observed in small HCC of the distinctly nodular type, which is usually moderately differentiated and encapsulated, even when the mass is

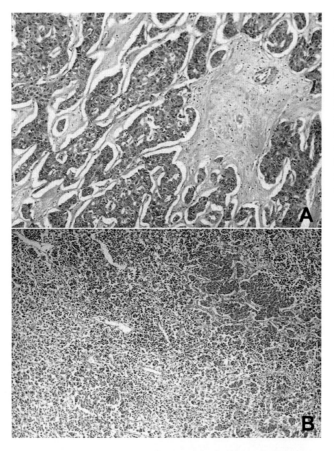

Figure 2.9 Histological variations in HCC. (a) Scirrhous type: fibrous connective tissue replaces the blood spaces and tumor cell nests are atrophic. (b) Sarcomatoid change: a tumor consists of a diffuse proliferation of short spindle-shaped sarcomatous cells, and transitional features from trabecular HCC (upper right) are observed in some cases. See color plate section.

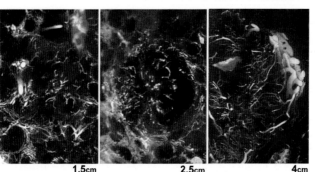

Figure 2.10 Angioarchitecture in HCC. The development of arterial tumor vessels parallels tumor growth, and portal veins (shown in blue) stay along the capsule when the tumor is encapsulated. See color plate section.

small. This remarkable difference in the development of the arterial tumor vessels explains why the vaguely nodular small HCC is hypovascular and the distinctly nodular is hypervascular, as shown in Figure 2.2. The elastic fibers of arterial tumor vessels appear sparse and indistinct, unlike the distinctly visible elastic fibers of normal arteries. The lack of a distinct layer of elastic fibers in arterial tumor vessels suggests that they are functionally different from normal arteries [33].

Venous tumor vessels

Venous tumor vessels have a thin wall without smooth muscle. Connections between dilated sinusoidal blood spaces and venous tumor vessels are frequently observed, and they are also connected to portal veins within and/or around the fibrous capsule, forming an important part of the drainage system of HCC.

Portal veins

Portal veins do not enter the tumor tissue in advanced HCC. Portal veins in the tumor capsule contribute to the venous drainage of the tumor. Postmortem angioarchitectural studies have demonstrated that the veins along the tumor capsule are filled by colored fluid injected via the portal vein at autopsy [52]. Dynamic CT studies have also shown that the portal veins around the tumor border contribute to venous drainage. This confirms that the portal veins around the tumor are the main drainage vessels in advanced HCC [53].

Sinusoid-like blood spaces

The stroma of HCC is largely composed of sinusoidal blood spaces mimicking the sinusoids in normal liver tissue. The characteristics of these spaces are different in advanced HCC and early-stage HCC. The spaces are lined by a single layer of endothelial cells, which are immunohistochemically positive to anti-CD34 antibody and anti-Factor-VIII-related antigen in advanced HCC. Since the endothelial cells of the sinusoids of normal liver are negative to these antibodies, the sinusoid-like blood spaces in advanced HCC are similar to capillaries, and these findings are called "capillarization" or "neovascularization" [34,53,54]. The degree of sinusoidal capillarization is closely related to the histological grade. Complete capillarization is seen mainly in moderately differentiated tumor, whereas in early-stage well-differentiated HCC capillarization is incomplete.

Pathology of metastatic liver cancers

Incidence

Metastatic liver cancer is far more frequent than primary liver cancer. In a large series of 19 208 autopsies of malignant extrahepatic tumors, Craig *et al.* [55] observed that hepatic metastases were 18 times commoner than primary malignant tumors. Pickren *et al.* [56] reported that metastatic liver tumors were 41 times more frequent than primary hepatic tumor in a large autopsy series. In Asian countries, where primary liver cancer is more frequent than in Western countries, metastases are more common than primary tumors, but the discrepancy in their occurrence is less marked. According to the Annual Registration of Pathological Autopsy Cases in Japan in 2002, there were 5504 (32.2%) metastases in a total of 17 085 malignant tumors.

Craig *et al.* [55] reported that lung, colon, pancreas, breast, and stomach were the most common sites of primary tumors in 1151 autopsy cases of metastatic liver cancers in the USA. Similar findings were observed in the 5504 autopsy cases of metastatic liver cancers in the Annual Registration of Pathological Autopsy Cases in Japan in 2002.

The frequency of hepatic metastases in cirrhotic and non-cirrhotic livers

It is a matter of controversy whether metastases occur less frequently in cirrhotic liver than in non-cirrhotic liver. Lisa *et al.* [57] described the rarity of metastasis in cirrhotic liver and postulated that it may be related to the infrequent association of cirrhosis and extrahepatic metastasis. Gall [58] reported metastases in 1% of cirrhotic livers in autopsy series, but their overall incidence in all livers examined at autopsy was 10%. Melato *et al.* [59] compared the frequency of hepatic metastasis in 5241 consecutive autopsies performed in Italy and 6511 autopsies in Japan, and found a decreased frequency of hepatic metastases in cirrhotic livers in both countries. On the other hand, Fisher *et al.* [60] found no statistically significant difference in the incidence of hepatic metastases in cirrhotic and non-cirrhotic patients. They suggested that a significant number of cirrhotics probably fail to achieve a sufficient span of life to develop extrahepatic carcinomas, because the mean age of cirrhotics without extrahepatic carcinomas at the time of death was significantly younger than that of cirrhotics with hepatic metastases.

Gross appearance of metastatic tumors

Most metastatic liver cancers present as multiple nodules of varying sizes; solitary metastases or confluent masses are relatively rare. Metastases to the liver were found in 39% in a series of 8455 autopsies of malignant tumors, and only 6% were solitary [55]. Necrosis is frequently observed, because of insufficient blood supply to the center of the tumor. Metastatic tumors located close to the liver capsule show a characteristic central depression described as "umbilication" (Fig. 2.11). In general,

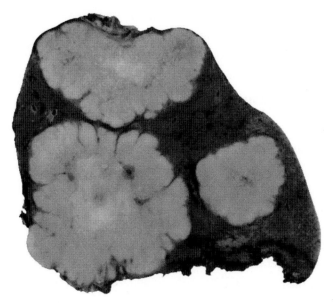

Figure 2.11 Metastasis of breast cancer. Metastatic tumors show central necrosis, and a tumor close to the liver capsule shows the characteristic depression called an "umbilication." *See color plate section.*

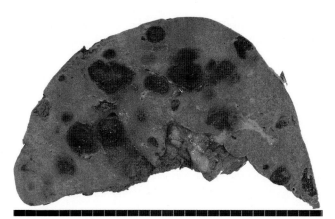

Figure 2.12 Metastasis of angiosarcoma. Multiple metastatic tumors are dark reddish in color, and metastasis of angiosarcoma can be predicted from the gross appearance. *See color plate section.*

the development of arteries in metastatic liver tumors is poor, especially in the central area of the mass, and it frequently causes central or generalized necrosis. Tumor thrombi in portal and hepatic veins, which are common in hepatocellular carcinoma, are rare in hepatic metastases. Hepatic metastases tend to exhibit the macroscopic characteristics of the primary tumor. For example, hepatic metastases from malignant melanoma, angiosarcoma, and liposarcoma show black, hemorrhagic red, and yellow color, respectively (Fig. 2.12). Thus it is often easy to specify the primary tumor on gross examination, based on the characteristic appearance of the metastases. A liver containing metastases from breast carcinoma, which has been repeatedly treated with chemotherapy, may present a coarsely lobulated appearance mimicking the "hepar lobatum" seen in syphilis [61].

Biopsy diagnosis of hepatic metastasis

On biopsy, it is frequently difficult to differentiate metastatic adenocarcinoma from intrahepatic cholangiocarcinoma when the hepatic tumor is solitary and there is no clinical manifestation of extrahepatic disease. Rullier *et al.* [62] reported that immunohistochemical analysis of cytokeratin (CK) 7 and 20 allows intrahepatic cholangiocarcinoma to be distinguished from metastatic colorectal adenocarcinoma. They demonstrated that cholangiocarcinoma is positive for CK7 and CK20 in 96% and 70%, respectively, and that the labeling index is high for CK7 but low or moderate for CK20. Many metastatic colorectal adenocarcinomas (81%) are negative for CK7, but all are positive for CK20, with a high labeling index. Hepatic metastases from tumors histologically mimicking HCC, such as renal cell carcinoma of the clear-cell type, clear-cell carcinoma of the female genital organs, adrenal carcinoma, hepatoid adenocarcinoma, epithelioid hemangioendothelioma, and carcinoid tumor, are also often problematic in biopsy diagnosis (Fig. 2.12) [33].

REFERENCES

1. Kondo Y, Niwa Y, Akikusa B, *et al.* A histopathologic study of early hepatocellular carcinoma. *Cancer* 1983; **52**: 687–92.
2. Okuda K. Early recognition of hepatocellular carcinoma. *Hepatology* 1986; **9**: 751–5.
3. Wada K, Kondo Y, Kondo F. Large regenerative nodules and dysplastic nodules in cirrhotic livers: a histopathologic study. *Hepatology* 1988; **8**: 1684–8.
4. Kondo F, Wada K, Nagato Y, *et al.* Biopsy diagnosis of well-differentiated hepatocellular carcinoma based on new morphologic criteria. *Hepatology* 1989; **9**: 751–5.
5. Takayama T, Makuuchi M, Hirohashi S, *et al.* Malignant transformation of adenomatous hyperplasia to hepatocellular carcinoma. *Lancet* 1990; **336**: 1150–3.
6. Sakamoto M, Hirohashi S, Shimosato Y. Early stages of multistep hepatocarcinogenesis: adenomatous hyperplasia and early hepatocellular carcinoma. *Hum Pathol* 1991; **22**: 172–8.
7. Eguchi A, Nakashima O, Okudaira S, *et al.* Adenomatous hyperplasia in the vicinity of small hepatocellular carcinoma. *Hepatology* 1992; **15**: 843–8.
8. Theise ND, Schwartz M, Miller C, *et al.* Macroregenerative nodules and hepatocellular carcinoma in forty-four sequential adult liver explants with cirrhosis. *Hepatology* 1992; **16**: 949–55.

9. Ferrell L, Wright T, Lake J, *et al.* Incidence and diagnostic features of macroregenerative nodules vs. small hepatocellular carcinoma in livers. *Hepatology* 1992; **16**: 1372–81.

10. Furuya K, Nakamura M, Yamamoto Y, *et al.* Macroregenerative nodule of the liver: a clinico-pathological study of 345 autosy cases of chronic liver disease. *Cancer* 1993; **61**: 99–105.

11. Terada T, Terasaki S, Nakanuma Y. A clinicopathologic study of adenomatous hyperplasia of the liver in 209 consecutive cirrhotic livers examined by autopsy. *Cancer* 1993; **72**: 1551–6.

12. Nakashima O, Sugihara S, Kage M, Kojiro M. Pathomorphologic characteristics of small hepato-cellular carcinoma: a special reference to small hepatocellular carcinoma with indistinct margins. *Hepatology* 1995; **22**: 101–5.

13. Sherman M, Peltekian KM, Lee C. Screening for hepatocellular carcinoma in chronic carriers of hepatitis B virus: incidence and prevalence of hepatocellular carcinoma in a North American urban population. *Hepatology* 1995; **22**: 432–8.

14. Hytiroglou P, Theise ND, Schwartz M, *et al.* Macroregenerative nodules in a series of adult cirrhotic liver explants: issues of classification and nomenclature. *Hepatology* 1995; **21**: 703–8.

15. Le Bail B, Belleannee G, Bernard PH, *et al.* Adenomatous hyperplasia in cirrhotic livers: histolo-gical evaluation, cellular density, and proliferative activity of 35 lesions in the cirrhotic explants of 10 adult French patients. *Hum Pathol* 1995; **26**: 897–906.

16. Mion F, Grozel K, Boillot O, *et al.* Adult cirrhotic liver explants: precancerous lesions and undetected small hepatocellular carcinomas. *Gastroenterology* 1996; **111**: 1587–92.

17. Kojiro M, Nakashima O. Histopathologic evaluation of hepatocellular carcinoma with special reference to small early stage tumor. *Semin Liver Dis* 1999; **19**: 287–96.

18. Bruix J, Sherman M, Llovet JM, *et al.* Clinical management of hepatocellular carcinoma: consensus of the Barcelona 2000 EASL conference. *J Hepatol* 2000; **35**: 421–30.

19. Kutami R, Nakashima Y, Nakashima O, *et al.* Pathomorphologic study on the mechanism of fatty change in small hepatocellular carcinoma of humans. *J Hepatol* 2000; **33**: 282–9.

20. Hytiroglou P. Morphological changes of early human hepatocarcinogenesis. *Semin Liver Dis* 2004; **24**: 65–75.

21. Kojiro M, Roskams T. Early hepatocellular carcinoma and dysplastic nodules. *Semin Liver Dis* 2005; **25**: 133–47.

22. Libbrecht L, Desmet V, Roskams T. Preneoplastic lesions in human hepatocarcinogenesis. *Liver Int* 2005; **25**: 16–27.

23. International Working Party. Terminology of nodular lesions of the liver: recommendations of the World Congress of Gastroenterology Working Group. *Hepatology* 1995; **22**: 983–93.

24. Terada T, Nakanuma Y. Survey of iron-accumulative macroregenerative nodules in cirrhotic livers. *Hepatology* 1989; **5**: 851–4.

25. Aihara T, Noguchi S, Sasaki Y, *et al.* Clonal analysis of regenerative nodules in hepatitis C virus-induced liver cirrhosis. *Gastroenterology* 1994; **107**: 1805–11.

26. Paradis V, Laurendeau I, Vidaud M, *et al.* Clonal analysis of macronodules in cirrhosis. *Hepatology* 1998; **28**: 953–8.

27. Paradis V, Bieche I, Dargere D, *et al.* Molecular profiling of hepatocellular carcinomas (HCC) using a large-scale real-time RT-PCR approach: determination of a molecular diagnostic index. *Am J Pathol* 2003; **163**: 733–41.

28. Ochiai T, Urata Y, Yamano T, *et al.* Clonal expansion in evolution of chronic hepatitis to hepatocellular carcinoma as seen at an X-chromosome locus. *Hepatology* 2000; **30**: 615–21.

29. Dhillon D, Colombari R, Savage K, *et al.* An immunohistochemical study of the blood vessels within primary hepatocellular tumors. *Liver* 1992; **12**: 311–18.

30. Park YN, Yang CP, Fernandez GJ, *et al.* Neoangiogenesis and sinusoidal "capillarization" in dysplastic nodules of the liver. *Am J Surg Pathol* 1998; **22**: 656–62.

31. Arakawa M, Kage M, Sugihara S, *et al.* Emergence of malignant lesions within an adenomatous hyperplastic nodule in a cirrhotic liver: observation in five cases. *Gastroenterology* 1986; **101**: 198–208.

32. Ohno Y, Shiga J, Machinami R. A histopathological analysis of five cases of adenomatous hyperplasia containing minute hepatocellular carcinoma. *Acta Pathol Jpn* 1990; **40**: 267–78.

33. Kojiro M. *Pathology of Hepatocellular Carcinoma.* Oxford: Blackwell, 2006.

34. Nakashima Y, Nakashima O, Hsia CC, *et al.* Vascularization of small hepatocellular carcinomas: correlation with differentiation. *Liver* 1999; **19**: 12–18.

35. Tomizawa M, Kondo F, Kondo Y, *et al.* Growth patterns and invasion of small hepatocellular carcinoma. *Pathol Int* 1995; **4**: 352–8.

36. Nakano M, Saito A, Yamamoto M, *et al.* Stromal and blood vessel wall invasion in well-differentiated hepatocellular carcinoma. *Liver* 1997; **45**: 41–6.

37. Matsui O, Takashima T, Kadoya M, *et al.* Dynamic computed tomography during arterial portography: the most sensitive examination for small hepatocellular carcinoma. *J Comput Assist Tomogr* 1985; **9**: 19–24.

38. Kenmochi K, Sugihara S, Kojiro M. Relationship of histologic grade of hepatocellular carcinoma (HCC) to tumor size, and demonstration of tumor cells of multiple different grades in a single small HCC. *Liver* 1987; **7**: 18–26.

39. Eggel H. Über das primäre Carcinom der Leber. *Beitr Pathol Anat Allg Pathol* 1901; **30**: 506.

40. Kim H, Park C, Han KH, *et al.* Primary liver carcinoma of intermediate (hepatocyte–cholangiocyte) phenotype. *J Hepatol* 2004; **40**: 298–304.

41. Lee JS, Heo J, Libbrecht L, *et al.* A novel prognostic subtype of human hepatocellular carcinoma derived from hepatic progenitor cells. *Nat Med* 2006; **12**: 410–16.

42. Wu PC, Lai VC, Lau VK, *et al.* Classification of hepatocellular carcinoma according to hepatocellular and biliary markers: clinical and biological implications. *Am J Pathol* 1996; **149**: 1167–75.

43. Aishima S, Nishida Y, Kuroda Y, *et al.* Histologic characteristics and prognostic significance in small hepatocellular carcinoma with biliary differentiation. *Am J Surg Pathol* 2007; **31**: 783–91.

44. Craig JR, Peters RL, Edmondson HA, *et al.* Fibrolamellar carcinoma of the liver: a tumor of adolescents and young adults with distinct clinicopathologic features. *Cancer* 1989; **46**: 372–9.

45. Stromeyer FW, Ishak KG, Gerber MA, *et al*. Ground-glass cells in hepatocellular carcinoma. *Am J Clin Pathol* 1980; **74**: 254–8.

46. Nakashsima O, Sugihara S, Eguchi A, *et al*. Pathomorphologic study of pale bodies in hepatocellular carcinoma. *Acta Pathol Jpn* 1992; **42**: 414–18.

47. Kurogi M, Nakashima O, Miyaaki H, *et al*. Clinicopathological study of scirrhous hepatocellular carcinoma. *J Gastroenterol Hepatol* 2006; **21**: 1470–77.

48. Yamaguchi R, Nakashima O, Yano H, *et al*. Hepatocellular carcinoma with sarcomatous change: a clinicopathological and immunohistochemical study of 6 surgical cases. *Oncol Rep* 1997; **4**: 525–9.

49. Kakizoe S, Kojiro M, Nakashima T. Hepatocellular carcinoma with sarcomatous change: clinicopathologic and immunohistochemical studies of 14 autopsy cases. *Cancer* 1987; **59**: 310–16.

50. Maeda T, Adachi E, Kajiyama K, *et al*. Spindle cell hepatocellular carcinoma: a clinicopathologic and immunohistochemical analysis of 15 cases. *Cancer* 1995; **77**: 51–7.

51. Haratake J, Horie A. An immunohistochemical study of sarcomatoid liver carcinomas. *Cancer* 1991; **68**: 93–7.

52. Nakashima T, Kojiro M. *Hepatocellular Carcinoma: an Atlas of its Pathology*. Tokyo: Springer-Verlag, 1987.

53. Ueda K, Matsui O, Kawamori Y, *et al*. Hypervascular hepatocellular carcinoma: evaluation of hemodynamics with dynamic CT during hepatic arteriography. *Radiology* 1998; **206**: 161–6.

54. Kin M, Torimura T, Ueno T, *et al*. Sinusoidal capillarization in small hepatocellular carcinoma. *Pathol Int* 1994; **44**: 771–8.

55. Craig JR, Peters RL, Edmondson HA. *Tumors of the Liver and Intrahepatic Bile Ducts. Atlas of Tumor Pathology*, 2nd series, 26. Washington, DC: Armed Forces Institute of Pathology, 1989.

56. Pickren JW, Tsukada Y, Lane WW. Liver metastases: analysis of autopsy data. In: Weiss L, Gilbert HA, eds. *Liver Metastasis*. Boston, MA: Hall Medical Publishers, 1982: 2–18.

57. Lisa JR, Solomon C, Gordon EJ. Secondary carcinoma in cirrhosis of liver. *Am J Pathol* 1942; **18**: 137–40.

58. Gall E. Primary and metastatic carcinoma of the liver: relationship to hepatic cirrhosis. *Arch Pathol* 1960; **70**: 226–32.

59. Melato M, Laurino L, Mucli E, *et al*. Relationship between cirrhosis, liver cancer, and hepatic metastases: an autopsy study. *Cancer* 1989; **64**: 455–9.

60. Fisher ER, Hellstrom HR, Fisher B. Rarity of hepatic metastasis in cirrhosis: a misconception. *JAMA* 1960; **174**: 366–9.

61. Qizilbash A, Kontozoglou T, Sianos J, Scully K. Hepar lobatum associated with chemotherapy and metastatic breast cancer. *Arch Pathol Lab Med* 1987; **111**: 58–61.

62. Rullier A, Le Bail B, Fawaz R, *et al*. Cytokeratin 7 and 20 expression in cholangiocarcinomas varies along the biliary tract but still differs from that in colorectal carcinoma metastases. *Am J Surg Pathol* 2000; **24**: 870–6.

3

Diagnostic imaging pre- and post-ablation

Chang-Hsien Liu, Kambadakone R. Avinssh, Debra A. Gervais, and Dushyant V. Sahani

Introduction

Hepatic malignant tumors are common worldwide. Surgical resection and, in rare instances, liver transplantation represent the gold standard of management, offering a chance of cure in selected patients [1,2]. The overall 3-year survival rate in patients with hepatocellular carcinoma (HCC) who undergo surgical resection is between 47.2% and 83.9% [3–5], and the overall 5-year survival rate in patients with colorectal liver metastases who undergo surgical resection is between 35% and 58% [6]. However, curative resection is frequently precluded because of medical comorbidities that render patients inoperable. Less than 25% of patients with either primary HCC or colorectal liver metastases are candidates for surgical resection [1,2].

Since the 1990s, radiofrequency ablation (RFA) of primary and secondary hepatic malignancies has had promising results in local control of tumors [7]. With advances in imaging modalities and refinements of ablation technique, as well as more powerful generators, the outcome of RFA for hepatic tumors has improved significantly in the past several years [3,4,8,9]. RFA can achieve complete necrosis of the tumor without adverse effects on liver function. To date, RFA is considered a reasonable alternative for patients with four or fewer hepatic tumors that are less than 3–5 cm in diameter. The absolute contraindications of RFA include extrahepatic disease, life expectancy less than 6 months, other active malignant disease, cirrhosis or hepatic insufficiency, portal hypertension or portal vein thrombosis, altered mental status, age less than 18 years, pregnancy, severe pulmonary disease, active infection, and refractory coagulopathy. The relative contraindications are tumors greater than 5 cm, more than four tumors, and tumors adjacent to large blood vessels, the pericardium, diaphragm, or other viscera [10].

Interventional Radiological Treatment of Liver Tumors, ed. Andy Adam and Peter R. Mueller.
Published by Cambridge University Press. © Cambridge University Press 2009.

It is therefore important to define tumor type, number, and location, and extra-hepatic metastases, on imaging for pre-ablation treatment planning.

However, incomplete treatment and local tumor progression after RFA remain clinical challenges [3,4,8,11–13]. It is important to detect residual or local tumor progression on imaging after treatment at an early stage so that an effective local therapy can be reinstituted. This chapter will focus on current clinical experience with imaging studies, including ultrasonography (US), computed tomography (CT), magnetic resonance imaging (MRI), integrated positron emission tomography (PET), and PET/CT, before and after liver RFA.

Imaging prior to liver ablation

Liver blood supply

There is a dual blood supply to the liver. The portal vein contributes up to 75–80% of hepatic blood flow, and the hepatic artery contributes the remaining 20–25% [14,15]. In contrast, hepatic neoplasms receive their blood supply primarily from the hepatic artery, with little or no supply from the portal vein [16]. Hepatic neoplasms may be classified as hypervascular or hypovascular, based on the degree of hepatic arterial blood supply or their enhancement pattern on the dynamic contrast-enhanced images [14]. Therefore, it is very important to evaluate the enhancement features of the hepatic neoplasms on imaging modalities for lesion detection and characterization.

Role of dynamic imaging

As a result of the liver's dual blood supply, triphase contrast-enhanced imaging of the liver is often performed, with the phases defined in relation to the moment when contrast medium arrives in the liver. The hepatic arterial phase of liver enhancement occurs 20–30 seconds after the start of an intravenous bolus of contrast medium. During this phase of enhancement, hypervascular hepatic neoplasms will be maximally enhanced, whereas the hepatic parenchyma will be only mini-mally enhanced, as three-quarters of hepatic parenchymal vascular supply is derived from portal venous blood, which at this point in the injection has not yet been replaced by contrast medium [16]. Hypovascular lesions are poorly imaged, due to reduced uptake of the contrast agent from the hepatic artery, and are hence hypointense in the arterial phase [14]. Therefore, identification of contrast enhancement patterns during the arterial phase is crucial for characterization of hypervascular hepatic lesions [14].

The phase of portal venous dominance, during which the hepatic parenchyma is maximally enhanced, occurs approximately 60–90 seconds after the start of a 2–3 ml s^{-1} IV contrast bolus. The relative delay in portal venous versus hepatic arterial enhancement is due to the additional time required for the contrast medium to pass through the mesentery and the spleen before entering the portal venous system [16]. During this portal venous phase the distinction between normal liver tissue and hypervascular lesions is lost, while hypovascular lesions become clearly visible as areas that are hypointense to normal tissue.

The equilibrium-phase image obtained after several minutes, when contrast medium has been eliminated from normal liver tissue, is useful to demonstrate persistent enhancement of some neoplasms (e.g., hemangiomas) and fibrotic lesions.

The degree of hepatic enhancement is determined by a combination of factors. The most important technique-related factors include contrast medium volume and concentration, rate of injection, and type of injection (i.e., uniphasic versus biphasic) [16]. In arterial-phase images, improved lesion-to-liver contrast can be achieved either by an accelerated injection rate (Fig. 3.1) or by an increased iodine concentration. While the injection rate of contrast medium (3–6 ml s^{-1}) may be physiologically limited, the case for using contrast agents with higher iodine

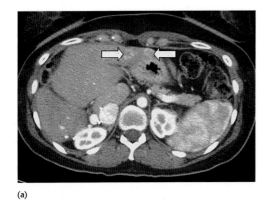
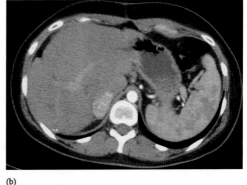

(a)   (b)

Figure 3.1 Improved detection of hepatocellular carcinoma (HCC) by an accelerated injection rate.
(a) Axial contrast-enhanced CT image in the arterial phase obtained with contrast injection rate of 3.5 ml s^{-1} shows two well-enhancing small nodules in segment II. (b) Axial contrast-enhanced CT image in the arterial phase with contrast injection rate of 2.5 ml s^{-1} does not show any enhancing nodules in the same location.

concentration (350–400 mg ml^{-1}) is compelling. Itoh *et al.* [17] and Awai *et al.* [18] showed improved arterial enhancement with contrast agents having high iodine concentration. However, in portal-venous-phase images, the degree of hepatic enhancement is directly proportional to the total amount of iodine administered.

Pre-RFA evaluation of hepatic lesions

Detection and characterization of hepatic lesions often presents a diagnostic challenge to the radiologist [14]. The objectives of liver imaging for pre-RFA treatment planning are the detection of hepatic lesions, the characterization of hepatic lesions, staging of neoplasms, the evaluation of biliary ductal status, and the assessment of vascular anatomy. It is important to understand the utility of various imaging modalities to optimally address the clinical question at hand.

Ultrasound (US) is an inexpensive and easily available imaging test for the evaluation of hepatic lesions. It is an excellent test to screen the liver for biliary obstruction or gallbladder disease, and to assess vascular patency. It is highly sensitive in differentiating a cyst from a solid hepatic lesion. However, routine transabdominal US is not as sensitive as CT or MRI for the detection and characterization of hepatic lesions [14]. The main limitations of US are high operator dependency, inability to detect lesions less than 1 cm in size, and low specificity [15,19]. The recent addition of US contrast media (not yet approved in the United States) for imaging the liver has shown promise in the characterization of various hepatic tumors [15,20]. Studies have shown accurate diagnosis of hepatic masses with contrast-enhanced ultrasonography (CEUS), according to the different contrast enhancements [19,21] (Table 3.1). In recent studies Quaia *et al.* [21] and Wilson *et al.* [19] have investigated the role of CEUS for the characterization of focal hepatic masses and have demonstrated an overall diagnostic accuracy of 82–86% as compared to 45–50% with conventional US. Recently, Janica *et al.* [22] demonstrated an increased diagnostic confidence for the detection and characterization of hepatic lesions with CEUS in comparison to dual-phase CT.

CT is the most frequently used imaging modality for the preoperative depiction of focal hepatic lesions. The use of a dual-phase helical CT technique with imaging during both the arterial and the portal venous phases of enhancement is particularly important in improving the depiction of hypervascular hepatic lesions [23] (Figs. 3.2 and 3.3). Multidetector-row computed tomography (MDCT), introduced in 1998, was a milestone in the development of CT technology [24]. MDCT provides short scan duration (a chest-to-pelvis examination is now possible in

Table 3.1 Diagnostic criteria for focal liver masses on CEUS

Lesion	CEUS criteria
Malignant	
HCC	Diffuse enhancement during arterial phase that decreases during portal venous and late phases, hypoechoic appearance
Metastasis	Enhancing peripheral rim, variable intralesional enhancement during arterial phase that decreases during portal venous and late phases, hypoechoic appearance
Benign	
Hemangioma	Nodular peripheral enhancement during arterial phase, with centripetal progression during portal venous and late phases
Focal nodular hyperplasia	Central spoke wheel-shaped enhancement during early arterial phase that becomes homogeneous during late arterial phase, homogeneous enhancement similar to that of the liver parenchyma during portal venous and late phases, hypoechoic central region corresponding to scar during late phase
Hepatocellular adenoma	Diffuse homogeneous or heterogeneous enhancement during arterial phase, enhancement similar to that of the liver parenchyma during portal venous and late phases, homogeneous or heterogeneous

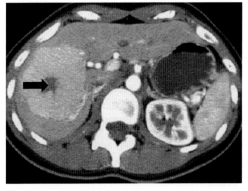 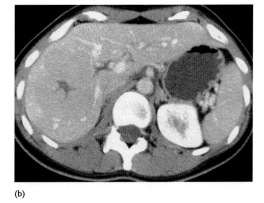

(a)　　　　　　　　　　　　　　　　　　　(b)

Figure 3.2 Focal nodular hyperplasia in a 30-year-old woman with upper abdominal pain.
(a) Axial contrast-enhanced CT image in the arterial phase shows a well-enhancing lesion with central scar (arrow) in the right lobe of the liver. (b) In the portal-venous phase, the lesion becomes isoattenuating to the liver while the central scar remains hypoattenuating.

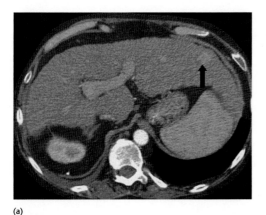
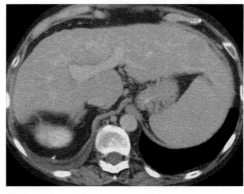

(a)   (b)

Figure 3.3 Hepatocellular carcinoma (HCC) in a 40-year-old woman with elevated AFP levels. (a) Axial contrast-enhanced CT image in the arterial phase shows an enhancing nodule (arrow) in the lateral segment of the left lobe of the liver. (b) In the portal-venous phase, the lesion is hypoattenuating to the liver, suggesting early contrast washout compared with liver parenchyma.

5–20 seconds) and high-resolution diagnostic images, and facilitates the generation of three-dimensional displays. With faster scanners, survey of multiple body parts can be undertaken in a single breath-hold, and the images are devoid of movement artifacts. It is also possible to routinely acquire near-isotropic data that result in esthetically pleasing two-dimensional (2D) and three-dimensional (3D) displays.

The advantages of MDCT can be exploited to the benefit of hepatobiliary imaging, for improved lesion detection, for multiplanar reconstruction, and for high-quality CT angiography. Recently, with the advent of 40–64-row detector scanners, the liver can be scanned with submillimeter collimation in a short breath-hold of not more than 5–8 seconds. This has enabled us to perform multiphase scanning of the liver during the optimal vascular phases, offering real arterial, portal venous, and equilibrium phases to characterize different kinds of hepatic tumors. Additionally, a marked decrease in slice thickness enables us to provide pretreatment isotropic and three-dimensional images of lesions in their precise anatomic locations. The typical MDCT protocol for the liver is shown in Table 3.2.

The advantages of MDCT for pre-RFA treatment planning of hepatic malignancy lie in accurate detection of the number of lesions and their location, in detecting extrahepatic spread of the tumor, and in mapping liver vascular anatomy. However, to minimize the radiation dose to the patient with MDCT, it is prudent to choose protocols with the phase of enhancement most appropriate for the indications. The indications for acquisition of multiphasic images are shown in Table 3.3.

Table 3.2 MDCT liver protocols on different CT scanners

Parameters	4 channel	16 channel	64 channel
Detector collimation (mm)	4×1.25	16×0.625	64×0.6
Table speed (mm s^{-1})	15	18.75	38
Pitch	1.0–2.0	0.938	0.984
Slice thickness (mm)			
Arterial phase (liver)	2.5–5.0	2.5	2.5
Venous phase (liver)	5.0	5.0	5.0
Scan delay to initiate arterial phase	Bolus tracking/automated trigger at 150 HU aortic enhancement followed by 10 seconds diagnostic delay. Empirical delay: 25–30 seconds		
Venous delay (s)	65–70	60	50–60

Table 3.3 Indications for acquisition of multiphase images in MDCT

Phase	Indications
Noncontrast	Diagnosis of fatty liver
	Diagnosis of hemorrhage
	Baseline for detection of calcification or confirmation of enhancement
Early arterial (arterographic)	CT arteriogram for arterial anatomy
20-second delay	Detection of hypervascular liver tumors
Late arterial (parenchymal arterial)	Detection of hypervascular liver tumors
40-second delay	Characterization of small lesions
Portal venous	Routine study
60–110-second delay	Liver metastases
Delayed (equilibrium), 2–15-minute delay	Diagnosis of cholangiocarcinoma, hemangioma

The multiplanar reformations and 3D display of the CT dataset provide an accurate relationship between the masses, hepatic vessels, bile ducts, and adjacent vital organs to facilitate RFA treatment planning (Fig. 3.4). It can help to achieve sufficient post-ablation margins and prevent local tumor progression and complication after RFA.

MRI has established its role as a preferred imaging modality for the detection and characterization of hepatic tumors. The technical advances achieved by MRI in

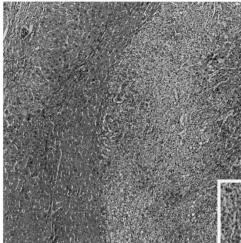

Fig. 2.1a
Dysplastic nodule. Low-grade dysplastic nodule: a nodule (right half) shows mildly increased cell density and clearer trabecular arrangement in parts.

Fig. 2.1b High-grade dysplastic nodule: a nodule (left half) shows markedly increased cell density with an irregular trabecular arrangement and fatty change.

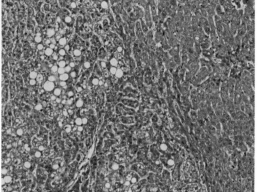

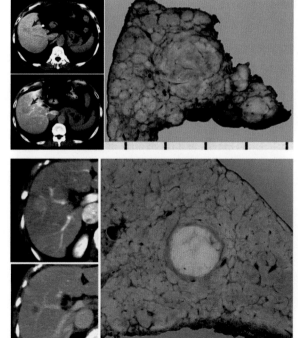

Fig. 2.2a
Small HCC. Vaguely nodular type: a tumor measuring 1.7 × 1.5 cm is vaguely nodular and retained portal tracts are recognizable; it is hypovascular on contrast CT.

Fig. 2.2b
Distinctly nodular type: a tumor of 1.2 cm in diameter is distinctly nodular and well encapsulated. On contrast CT, a tumor shows hypervascularity and "wash-out" as seen in classical HCC.

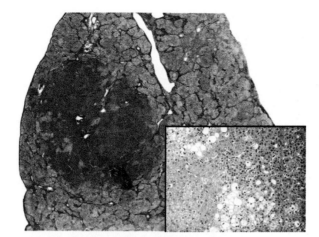

Fig. 2.3
Histological findings of vaguely nodular small HCC. The tumor consists of uniformly distributed well-differentiated HCC tissue with retained portal tracts, and shows a replacing growth at the tumor boundary without forming a capsule (inset).

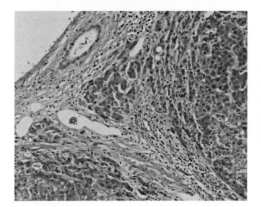

Fig. 2.4
"Stromal invasion" in well-differentiated HCC of the vaguely nodular type. This tumor-cell infiltration into the portal tract within the tumor is a helpful morphologic clue in distinguishing well-differentiated HCC from high-grade DN.

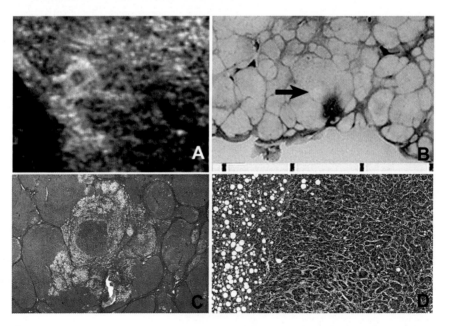

Fig. 2.5
A "nodule-in-nodule" appearance in early-stage HCC. (a) On ultrasound, a tumor shows a hypoechoic subnodule within a hyperechoic tumor. (b) Grossly, a tumor measuring 1 cm in diameter contains a minute whitish nodule (arrow). (c, d) Histologically, an outer nodule consists of well-differentiated HCC with fatty change, and a subnodule consists of moderately differentiated HCC without fatty change.

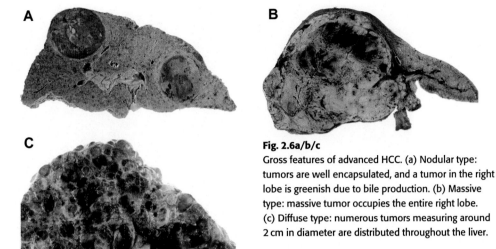

Fig. 2.6a/b/c
Gross features of advanced HCC. (a) Nodular type: tumors are well encapsulated, and a tumor in the right lobe is greenish due to bile production. (b) Massive type: massive tumor occupies the entire right lobe. (c) Diffuse type: numerous tumors measuring around 2 cm in diameter are distributed throughout the liver.

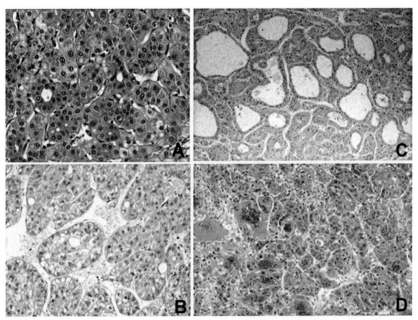

Fig. 2.7
Histologic features of HCC. (a) Well-differentiated: irregular thin trabecular pattern with occasional pseudoglands is characteristic. (b) Moderately differentiated: tumor shows varying sized tumor-cell islands (trabeculae) as if they are floating in sinusoidal blood spaces. (c) Pseudoglandular type: varying sized pseudoglands containing protein-like fluid are frequently observed in moderately differentiated HCC, and HCC with a prominent pseudoglandular pattern is called pseudoglandular type. (d) Poorly differentiated: tumor consists of mononuclear and/or multinuclear bizarre giant cells with a vague trabecular or solid pattern, and it is also called giant-cell HCC.

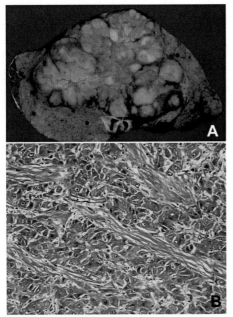

Fig. 2.8

Fibrolamellar carcinoma. (a) Gross appearance: tumor shows a central fibrous scar with radiating fibrous bands dividing the tumor into lobules, mimicking focal nodular hyperplasia. (b) Histologically, the tumor cells have abundant and deeply eosinophilic cytoplasm with round nuclei having distinct nucleoli. The tumor grows in sheets or small trabeculae, which are separated by fibrous collagen with a characteristic lamellar pattern.

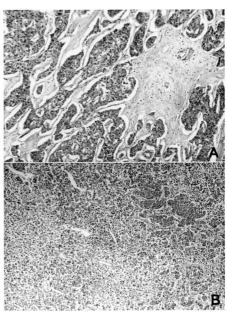

Fig. 2.9

Histological variations in HCC. (a) Scirrhous type: fibrous connective tissue replaces the blood spaces and tumor cell nests are atrophic. (b) Sarcomatoid change: a tumor consists of a diffuse proliferation of short spindle-shaped sarcomatous cells, and transitional features from trabecular HCC (upper right) are observed in some cases.

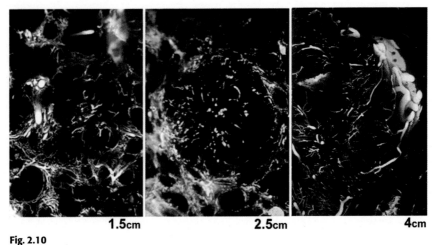

1.5cm   **2.5**cm   **4**cm

Fig. 2.10

Angioarchitecture in HCC. The development of arterial tumor vessels parallels tumor growth, and portal veins (shown in blue) stay along the capsule when the tumor is encapsulated.

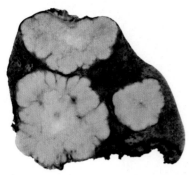

Fig. 2.11
Metastasis of breast cancer. Metastatic tumors show central necrosis, and a tumor close to the liver capsule shows the characteristic depression called an "umbilication."

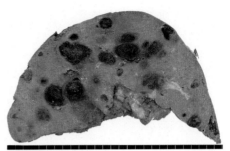

Fig. 2.12
Metastasis of angiosarcoma. Multiple metastatic tumors are dark reddish in color, and metastasis of angiosarcoma can be predicted from the gross appearance.

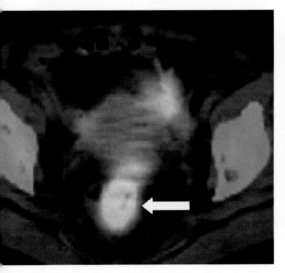

.6a

Fig. 3.6b

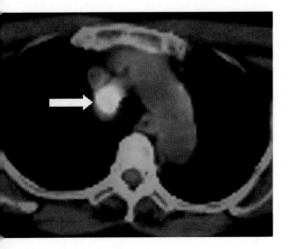

.6c

Fig. 3.6
Hybrid positron emission tomography/computed tomography (PET/CT) in a 71-year-old woman with a hepatic metastasis from rectal adenocarcinoma over segment I. (a) Axial image over the pelvis shows a segmental hypermetabolic area over the rectum (arrow), consistent with rectal adenocarcinoma. (b) Axial image over the liver shows a hypermetabolic lesion over segment I (arrow), consistent with hepatic metastasis. (c) Axial image also demonstrates a hypermetabolic nodule over the mediastinum (arrow), consistent with nodal metastasis.

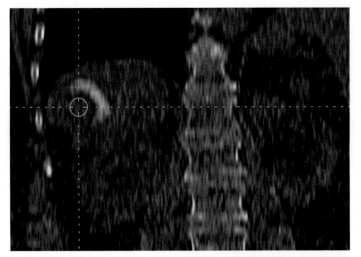

Fig. 3.16b
Coronal image also demonstrates a rim hypermetabolic area outside the prior treated area over segment IV, consistent with recurrence.

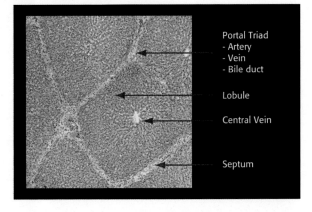

Fig. 5.2
Hematoxylin and eosin (H&E) stained section of porcine liver tissue showing normal structure of the liver.

Portal Triad
- Artery
- Vein
- Bile duct

Lobule

Central Vein

Septum

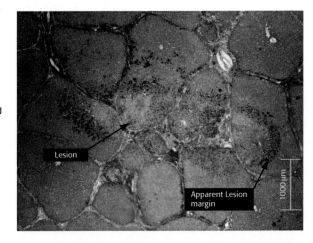

Fig. 5.3
Hematoxylin and eosin stain of a HIFU lesion in perfused porcine liver. The lesion is enclosed within the hemorrhagic rim (× 20).

Lesion

Apparent Lesion margin

1000 μm

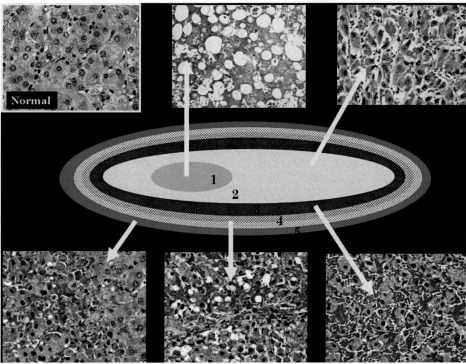

Fig. 5.4
Schematic of a HIFU lesion stained with hematoxylin and eosin (× 200 magnification). The different bands of tissue destruction referred to in the text may be seen. (1) Central region, showing most distinct damage and regions lacking cellular structure. (2) Region showing less intense staining, and increased extracellular spacing. (3) Hemorrhagic rim. (4) Region which overlaps regions 3 and 5 and contains "holes." (5) Region in which some hepatocyte nuclei appear condensed.

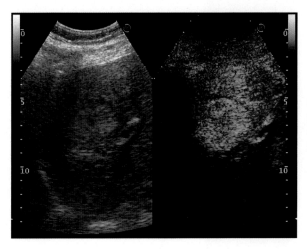

Fig. 8.3b
Dual ultrasound imaging (left, baseline; right, contrast-enhanced) confirms hypervascular tumor.

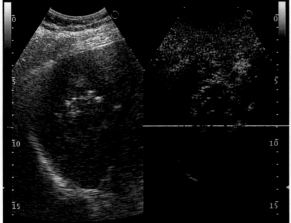

Fig. 8.3c
Dual ultrasound imaging repeated at the end of the procedure shows non-enhancing ablation zone with periablational enhancement. Follow-up computed tomography images obtained in.

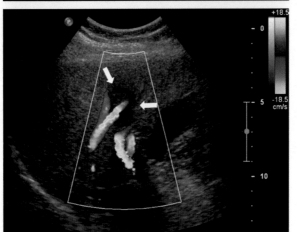

Fig. 10.1b
Color Doppler image prior to cryoablation identifying brisk flow within the hepatic venous branch coursing through the hypoechoic lesion (arrows).

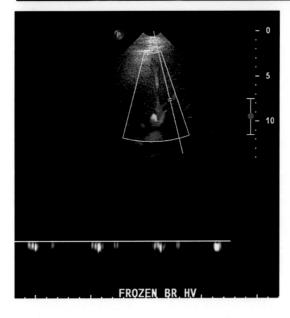

Fig. 10.1c
Color and pulsed Doppler image during cryoablation shows some probable transmitted pulsations, but no real flow within the more proximal hepatic venous branch after the iceball had enveloped the mass and hepatic vein.

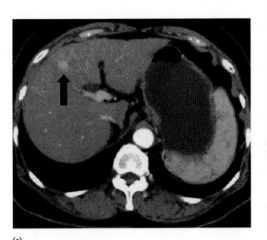
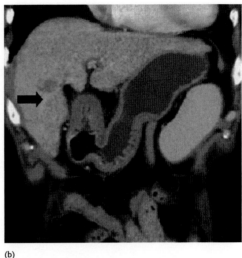

(a)   (b)

**Figure 3.4 Hepatocellular carcinoma (HCC) in a 59-year-old woman detected on 64-slice MDCT.
(a) Axial contrast-enhanced CT image in the arterial phase shows an intensely enhancing nodule (arrow)
in segment V of the liver. (b) Coronal reformatted image in the portal-venous phase clearly demonstrates
the lesion in close proximity to the middle hepatic vein (arrow). The multiplanar reformations provide
information crucial for RFA treatment planning.**

recent years have improved the anatomic coverage, image quality, and spatial resolution, to the benefit of liver imaging. One of the major advantages of MRI over other imaging modalities is the superior soft-tissue contrast, which allows easier characterization of focal hepatic lesions. In addition, two different groups of MRI contrast media for liver imaging are available: the non-specific gadolinium chelates and the liver-specific MRI contrast media. The latter group can be divided into two subgroups, the hepatobiliary contrast media and the reticuloendothelial (or Kupffer cell) contrast media [25]. Appropriate use of these agents, based on the clinical indications, can improve the accuracy of detection and characterization of focal hepatic lesions.

More importantly, MRI facilitates characterization of even subcentimeter focal hepatic lesions, a common occurrence on imaging in patients undergoing screening or oncologic survey exam. Routine use of advanced CT techniques, especially MDCT, has further contributed to increased detection of such small hepatic lesions. These lesions may be benign or malignant, and therefore characterization of small focal hepatic lesions is critical in treatment decisions. These lesions are often interpreted as too small to characterize, or indeterminate, as the attenuation measurements of these lesions on CT can be unreliable because of partial volume

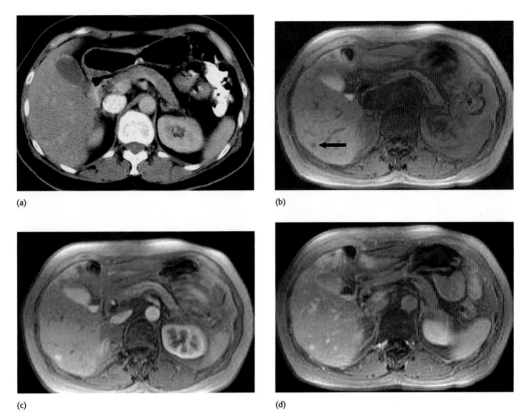

(a)

(b)

(c)

(d)

Figure 3.5 Improved characterization of a small hepatic lesion by contrast-enhanced MRI in a 45 year-old man. (a) Axial contrast-enhanced CT image in the portal-venous phase demonstrates a small faintly enhancing nodule in segment VI of the right lobe. Accurate diagnosis is not possible due to inadequate spatial resolution. (b) Pre-contrast T1-weighted MR image demonstrates the hypointense nodule in segment VI. (c) Contrast-enhanced T1-weighted image in the arterial phase shows intense enhancement within the lesion. (d) In the equilibrium phase, persistent enhancement is seen in the lesion, which is consistent with a hemangioma.

averaging and pseudo-enhancement. In patients with a history of a known cancer, small hepatic lesions discovered on imaging studies may require further evaluation to exclude a diagnosis of metastasis. Contrast-enhanced MRI can accurately characterize the majority of subcentimeter (< 10 mm) hepatic lesions (Fig. 3.5).

The standard MRI protocol for the hepatobiliary system is shown in Table 3.4. In a recent study, Holalkere *et al.* [26] have shown that MRI was 97.5% specific as compared to 77.3% for MDCT in hepatic mass characterization. Thus MRI performed after MDCT is justifiable for accurate characterization of subcentimeter focal hepatic lesions discovered on MDCT [26].

Table 3.4 MR liver protocols

Sequence	Parameters
Pre-contrast images	
Scout	T2 single shot fast spin echo in coronal plane
In-phase T1-weighted axial images	Gradient echo images (TE: approximately 2.1, 6.3, 10.5 ms at 1.5 T); 5–7 mm slice thickness
Out-phase T1-weighted axial images	Gradient echo images (TE: approximately 4.2, 8.4, 12.6 ms at 1.5 T); 5–7 mm slice thickness
Dual-echo T2-weighted axial images	Fast-spin-echo respiratory trigger with fat saturation; 5–8 mm slice thickness
Pre-contrast T1-weighted axial images	Gradient-echo out-phase with fat saturation; 5–7 mm slice thickness
Post-contrast images	Gadolinium 20 cm^3 with injection rate 2–3 cm^3 per second
Arterial phase	20-second post-gadolinium injection; T1-weighted gradient-echo images with fat saturation
Portal venous phase	60-second post-gadolinium injection; T1-weighted gradient-echo images with fat saturation
Equilibrium phase	180-second post-gadolinium injection; T1-weighted gradient-echo images with fat saturation

Screening for extrahepatic extension

It is important to detect extrahepatic tumor extension and nodal metastasis of hepatic malignancy for pre-RFA treatment planning, since extrahepatic disease is one of the absolute contraindications of RFA. 18-F-fluorodeoxyglucose positron emission tomography (FDG-PET) has not yet been established for pre-RFA evaluation. It can be used to exclude extrahepatic disease not evident on CT or MRI that may alter the planned RFA. Lai *et al.* [27] demonstrated previously unsuspected extrahepatic disease in 32% of patients with metastatic colorectal cancer scheduled for hepatic metastatectomy, predominantly involving the celiac lymph nodes. Desai *et al.* [28] also reported that FDG-PET showed extrahepatic disease in 72% of patients with metastatic colorectal cancer that was not found on CT. FDG-PET, as mentioned above, might assist in the accurate localization of extrahepatic disease.

The hybrid positron emission tomography/computed tomography (PET/CT) is a fusion technology that combines the advantages of both MDCT and PET scanning to offer not only anatomic details but also metabolic information about the

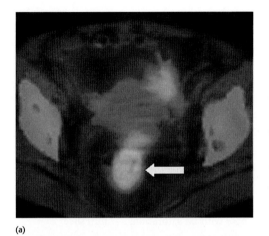

(a)

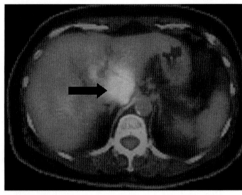

(b)

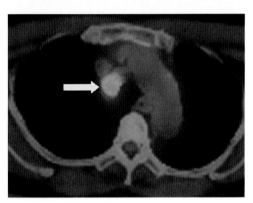

(c)

Figure 3.6 Hybrid positron emission tomography/ computed tomography (PET/CT) in a 71-year-old woman with a hepatic metastasis from rectal adenocarcinoma over segment I. (a) Axial image over the pelvis shows a segmental hypermetabolic area over the rectum (arrow), consistent with rectal adenocarcinoma. (b) Axial image over the liver shows a hypermetabolic lesion over segment I (arrow), consistent with hepatic metastasis. (c) Axial image also demonstrates a hypermetabolic nodule over the mediastinum (arrow), consistent with nodal metastasis. *See color plate section.*

pathologic process. PET/CT is now increasingly being used in oncology for the detection and staging of a wide variety of cancers [29–31]. It increases the accuracy of diagnosis compared with the individual PET and CT scans.

The advantages of PET/CT can therefore be utilized for detecting or ruling out extrahepatic tumor extension or nodal metastasis in selected patients who are being considered for RFA treatment for hepatic malignancy and are at risk for extrahepatic disease (Fig. 3.6). PET/CT can potentially detect the early changes (microinvasion) of surrounding liver tissue, to prevent local tumor progression after RFA. In addition, relying exclusively on macromorphological characteristics to make a conclusion runs the risk of misdiagnosis, mainly because of the intrinsic limitations of the conventional imaging modalities. PET/CT performed after other imaging modalities is justifiable for accurate tumor staging in patients who are at high risk for tumor metastases.

Imaging following liver ablation

Post-RFA change in liver tissue

Radiofrequency ablation refers to the induction of thermal injury due to frictional heat generated by the ionic agitation of particles within tissue following the application of alternating current. The frictional heat that occurs desiccates the surrounding tissue, leading to the evaporation of intercellular water and cellular disruption. The area of thermal injury of liver can be shaped according to the size, position, and shape of the electrode used [32,33]. The area of RF-induced coagulated tissue forms a necrotic scar that usually shrinks with time, but most often very slowly [34].

Imaging protocol for post-ablation follow-up

CT is the most frequently performed and widely used imaging modality in the early detection of residual or local tumor progression after RFA. The post-ablation CT scanning protocol typically follows the pretreatment protocol for consistency. Dynamic multiphasic imaging, including non-contrast, arterial, portal venous, and equilibrium phases, is needed to detect the viable tumor or tumor regrowth. The enhancing pattern of residual or recurrent tumor is influenced by lesion type.

Ninomiya *et al.* [35] recommend that dynamic CT using MDCT immediately after RFA is useful to evaluate the therapeutic effect. However, it may be very difficult to distinguish residual tumor from hyperemia induced by the ablation on images immediately after RFA. Our current practice is to recommend re-treatment for patients who have evidence of residual tumor based on a CT scan 1 month post-RFA.

Long-term imaging follow-up is necessary to ascertain the presence or absence of residual or recurrent tumor in the treated area, and a deep knowledge of time-related changes of the treated area and the surrounding normal parenchyma is important to assess the therapeutic response of hepatic tumors to RFA [36]. However, it is necessary to remember that the absence of contrast enhancement in the ablated lesion at short-term follow-up imaging after treatment (within 3 months) does not always indicate successful treatment, since later follow-up studies can demonstrate tumor regrowth at the periphery of the ablated lesion [36].

We currently obtain initial contrast-enhanced multiphase imaging for follow-up one month after RFA; the follow-up is at 3 months in the first year, and every 6 months thereafter [37]. Table 3.5 lists the salient features of the imaging findings

Table 3.5 Salient imaging findings following RFA of hepatic tumors

Category	CEUS	CT	MRI
Expected findings, indicative of successful treatment	Absence of vascularity on contrast-enhanced color or power Doppler US	1. Completely hypoattenuating tumor with no foci of enhancement within the lesion or in the periphery 2. Hyperdense areas within the lesion on unenhanced scans 3. Initial increase in size followed by decrease in size of lesion 4. Absent enhancement on post-contrast scans 5. Thin, regular, peripheral rim type of enhancement, high on portal-venous and equilibirium phase	1. Hyperintense on T1WI and hypointense on T2WI 2. Marked hyperintensity on T2WI in lesions with liquefactive necrosis 3. On contrast-enhanced T1WI, absent enhancement on all phases 4. Thin, regular, peripheral rim enhancement
Indeterminate findings		1. Ablated tumor not larger than pre-ablated tumor in the immediate scan 2. Marginal hypervascularity in the ablated zone (sometimes difficult to differentiate between residual tumor and arterioportal shunting or vascularized inflammatory reaction)	1. Marginal hypervascularity in the ablated zone (sometimes difficult to differentiate between residual tumor and arterioportal shunting or vascularized inflammatory reaction) 2. Marked hyperintensity in the event of liquefactive necrosis can sometimes be difficult to differentiate from tumor
Findings indicating residual or recurrent tumor	Focal flow signals within the tumor representing tumoral vascularity on contrast-enhanced power Doppler US	1. Nodular areas of enhancement within the lesion on the inner or outer side 2. Thick, irregular peripheral areas of enhancement 3. Enhancing areas are hypoattenuating to liver on portal-venous phase	1. Hyperintense areas within the tumor on T2WI 2. Nodular areas of enhancement within the tumor 3. Thick, irregular, peripheral areas of enhancement on post-contrast T1WI

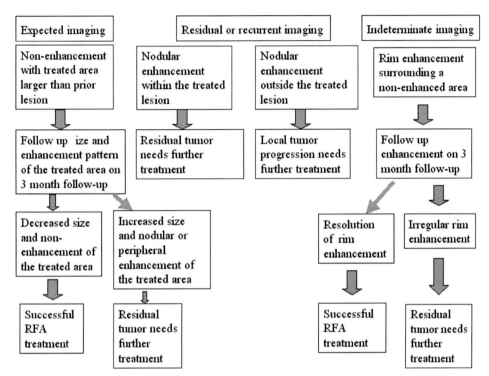

Figure 3.7 Flowchart depicting management strategies based on the imaging findings of focal hepatic tumor treated by RFA on 1-month follow-up MDCT.

on CEUS, MDCT, and MRI after RFA of hepatic tumors. The flowchart of differential diagnosis of focal hepatic tumors treated by RFA on 1-month follow-up imaging is shown in Figure 3.7.

Imaging findings after liver ablation

Expected imaging (complete ablation)

The success of RFA in hepatic malignancies is determined by the absence or presence of residual tumor. Complete ablation generates an area of thermocoagulation whose diameter is larger than or at least equivalent to that of the tumor.

On the non-enhanced post-RFA CT, an area of high density within the ablated region is an expected finding. It is thought that this area of high density is a

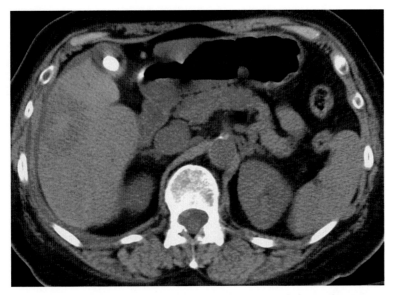

Figure 3.8 60-year-old woman with solitary hepatic metastasis from colon cancer on follow-up.
Axial unenhanced CT image obtained 1 month after RFA demonstrates high-density area within the
ablated region, consistent with thermocoagulated necrosis.

manifestation of greater cellular disruption, protein coagulation in the tissue, and
blood products [37] (Fig. 3.8). But non-enhanced CT is insensitive in the detection
of residual tumor tissue, due to poor soft-tissue contrast between the lesion and
zones of ablation. Successfully and completely ablated tumors do not demonstrate
contrast enhancement, because of complete tumor necrosis, and demonstrate a uniform low density on contrast-enhanced CT (Fig. 3.9). Complete non-enhancement
of the ablated lesions during all CT acquisition phases is considered evidence of
complete tumor necrosis at subsequent follow-up CT [37].

On MRI, most of the RF-treated lesions are hyperintense on T1-weighted images,
which is probably due to proteinaceous material or hemorrhage within the treated
lesion. Compared to the T1-weighted images, the RF-treated lesions usually appear
hypointense on T2-weighted images, and this hypointensity could be explained by
the dehydrating effect of RF-induced thermal damage, which results in coagulative
necrosis [34]. However, marked hyperintensity on T2-weighted images may also be
identified in some successfully treated lesions, and this marked hyperintensity could
signify a biloma or liquefactive necrosis, as active tumor always displays a less
heavily intense T2 signal intensity. On contrast-enhanced T1-weighted MR images,
the treated lesions show lack of enhancement from arterial to equilibrium phases,
indicative of complete efficient treatment (Fig. 3.10).

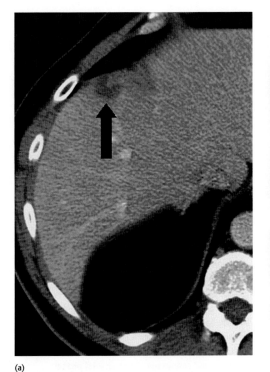

(a)

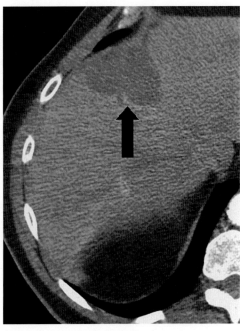

(b)

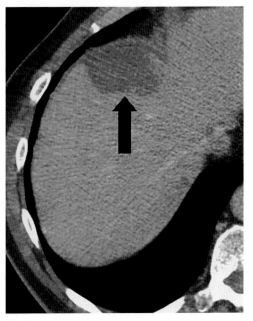

(c)

Figure 3.9 Follow-up CT images after successful RFA treatment in a 73-year-old man with a metastatic colon carcinoma. (a) Pre-RFA axial contrast-enhanced CT image in the portal-venous phase shows a low-density nodule (arrow) in segment IV, consistent with metastatic colon carcinoma. (b) Axial contrast-enhanced CT in the arterial phase obtained 3 months after RFA shows no contrast enhancement within the ablated area (arrow). (c) In the equilibrium phase, the ablated area does not demonstrate any enhancement (arrow). The absence of contrast enhancement indicates successful treatment without recurrence.

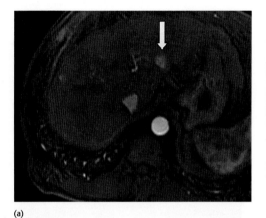

(a)

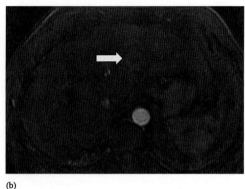

(b)

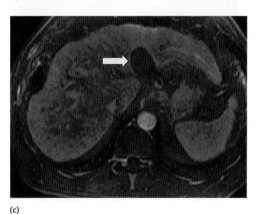

(c)

Figure 3.10 Follow-up MR images in a 55-year-old man with a hepatocellular carcinoma (HCC) after successful RFA treatment. (a) Pre-RFA contrast-enhanced fat-suppressed T1-weighted MR image in the arterial phase shows an intensely enhancing nodule (arrow) in the left lobe of the liver, consistent with hepatocellular carcinoma. (b) Contrast-enhanced fat-suppressed T1-weighted MR image in the arterial phase obtained 3 months after RFA shows no contrast enhancement within the ablated area (arrow). (c) In the equilibrium phase, the ablated area demonstrates no contrast enhancement (arrow), indicating complete necrosis of the HCC.

Filippone *et al.* [35] suggested that an immediate increase in the size of treated lesions within 1 month after RFA is a sign of correct performance of the procedure, since it ensures complete necrosis due to the ablation of the surrounding 0.5–1 cm of normal hepatic tissue. On long-term follow-up, all successfully treated lesions show a progressive reduction in size (Fig. 3.11). The non-enhancement of the treated lesions and progressive reduction in size of the ablative zones are considered to be the most reliable findings in successful ablation, and are indicative of complete tumor necrosis.

Multiplanar reformation (MPR) imaging of the liver offered by MDCT provides accurate demarcation between the zones of ablation and lesions for post-RFA evaluation. Coronal and sagittal MPR images facilitate the evaluation of therapeutic

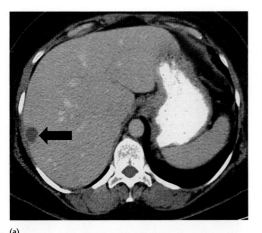

(a)

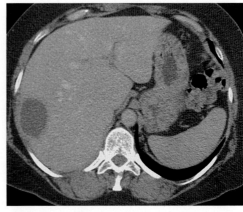

(b)

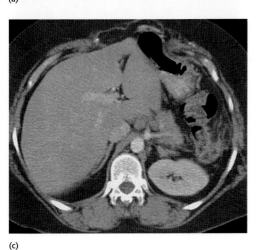

(c)

Figure 3.11 Follow-up CT images after successful RFA treatment of metastatic ovarian carcinoma in a 45-year-old woman. (a) Axial contrast-enhanced CT image obtained prior to RFA in the portal-venous phase shows a hypoattenuating nodule (arrow) in segment VI, consistent with metastatic ovarian carcinoma. (b) Axial contrast-enhanced CT image in the portal-venous phase obtained 1 month post RFA shows a large hypoattenuating area in the region of the ablated metastatic focus. (c) Axial contrast-enhanced CT image in the portal-venous phase obtained after 18 months of RFA shows complete resolution of the metastatic focus with no demonstrable lesion.

effect in lesions located at the liver dome or edge when adequate visualization is not possible with axial images alone [36].

Indeterminate imaging (needs follow-up)

It may be very difficult to distinguish residual tumor from hyperemia induced by ablation, and often accurate assessment can only be made after reviewing serial imaging scans. The thin, regular, peripheral rim type of enhancement seen at the end of 1 month is considered as congestion and/or granulation tissue secondary to RFA and is not indicative of a viable tumor, and it usually resolves on the

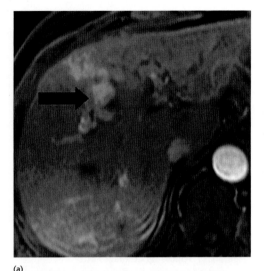

(a)

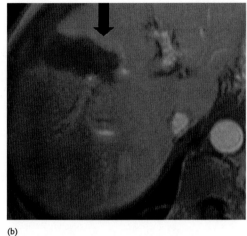

(b)

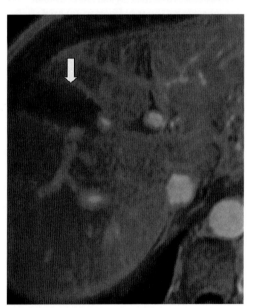

(c)

Figure 3.12 Pre- and post-RFA MR images in a 57-year-old man with a hepatocellular carcinoma (HCC). (a) Pre-RFA axial contrast-enhanced fat-suppressed MR image in the arterial phase shows an intensely enhancing nodular lesion in segment IV, consistent with HCC. (b) Contrast-enhanced T1-weighted MR image in the portal-venous phase 1 month after RFA shows a thin, regular, peripheral rim enhancement of the treated area (arrow), indicating congestion and/or granulation tissue. These MR features are considered indeterminate findings. (c) Contrast-enhanced T1-weighted MR image in the portal-venous phase obtained 3 months post RFA reveals near-complete resolution of the peripheral rim enhancement in the ablated area (arrow), indicating successful RFA treatment.

follow-up study at 3 months [35, 37–38] (Fig. 3.12). It has been shown by comparison with histologic findings that the thin ring is a vascularized inflammatory reaction with granulation tissue surrounding the zone of coagulation necrosis [39–42]. Reactive enhancement, independent of its shape (i.e., peripheral, wedge,

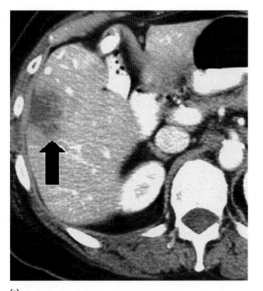

(a)

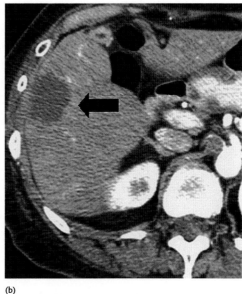

(b)

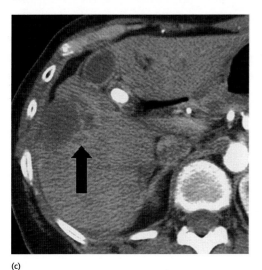

(c)

Figure 3.13 Indeterminate imaging findings in the follow-up CT images after RFA treatment in a 67-year-old woman with a hepatic metastasis from breast carcinoma.
(a) Pre-RFA axial contrast-enhanced CT in the arterial phase shows a hypoattenuating lesion (arrow) in segment V, consistent with metastasis. (b) Axial contrast-enhanced CT in the arterial phase after 1 month of RFA shows a thin, regular, peripheral rim enhancement of the treated area (arrow). (c) Axial contrast-enhanced CT image in the arterial phase obtained 3 months post RFA shows the progression of the peripheral rim enhancement into irregular and nodular areas, suggesting tumor recurrence (arrow).

or nodular) is never hypoattenuating in the portal and equilibrium phases, whereas the residual or recurrent neoplastic tissue is more often hypoattenuating during the equilibrium phase [35]. However, if the thin, regular, peripheral rim-type enhancement becomes thick and irregular with enhancement in the follow-up imaging, residual tumor with local progression should be considered and further treatment is needed (Fig. 3.13).

Another RF-induced modification is the presence, on arterial-phase images, of wedge-shaped enhancement in the liver parenchyma adjacent to the RF-treated area. This enhancement probably corresponds to peripheral arterioportal shunts caused either by the needle puncture and/or by thermal damage. These wedge-shaped areas should not be misinterpreted as tumor contrast-material uptake [34].

The thin, regular, peripheral rim-type enhancement and wedge-shaped enhancement of the treated lesion within 1 month of follow-up are not considered to be residual tumor and need imaging follow-up.

Residual and recurrent imaging

A residual tumor is determined by viable tumor within the treated lesion, and is often detected in the first post-RFA follow-up imaging. On the other hand, a recurrent tumor presents typically as new satellite lesions out of the treated lesion, or uncommonly as new tumor growth in the treated zone, and is detected in the subsequent follow-up imaging. On CT study, the residual or recurrent tumor appears as a hypoattenuating focus during the equilibrium phase in both HCC and metastatic nodules, its attenuation during the arterial and the portal-venous phases being influenced by lesion type. During the arterial phase residual tumor is hyperattenuating in HCC nodules and hypervascular metastases, whereas it is hypoattenuating in hypovascular metastatic lesions [36]. During the portal-venous phase, residual tumor is hypoattenuating in HCC nodules and hypervascular metastases, whereas it is also hypoattenuating in hypovascular metastatic lesions.

Lesion enhancement pattern is another important factor in evaluating therapeutic efficacy. The most common pattern of enhancement seen in unsuccessfully treated lesions is nodular. The nodular enhancement pattern of the inner border of treated lesion is present only in lesions with residual tumor seen within 1 month after RFA, whereas the nodular enhancement pattern of the outer border of treated lesions or other locations was present in lesions with recurrence observed 1 month after the procedure [36] (Fig. 3.14). The thick, irregular, peripheral rim-type enhancement is another enhancement pattern of the residual tumor at subsequent follow-up images.

Recently, MDCT has demonstrated several clearly distinct hepatic circulatory phases, including early arterial, arterial, portal-venous, and equilibrium phases, and has made detection of residual or recurrent lesions easier than with dual-phase CT.

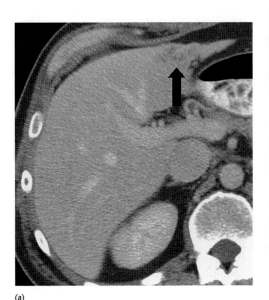

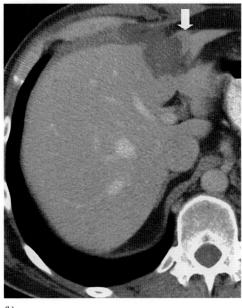

(a)   (b)

Figure 3.14 Post-RFA residual tumor in a 49-year-old man with a treated hepatic metastasis from esophageal carcinoma. (a) Pre-RFA axial contrast-enhanced CT image in the portal venous phase shows a lobulated heterogeneously enhancing low-density lesion (arrow) in segment IV, consistent with metastasis. (b) Post-RFA 1-month follow up axial contrast-enhanced CT image in the portal venous phase shows a persistent enhancing nodule in the region of ablation (arrow), indicating residual tumor.

On MRI, residual or recurrent tumors always show moderate (different from a fluid signal) hyperintensity on T2-weighted images, regardless of tumor type. On contrast-enhanced T1-weighted images, the residual tumors or recurrent tumors mostly show either nodular enhancement on arterial phase (HCCs or hypervascular hepatic metastases) or hypoattenuation on portal-venous phase (hypovascular hepatic metastases) (Fig. 3.15). Dromain *et al.* [34] reported that MRI depicted more local regrowth (8/9) than CT (4/9) but without significant differences. The higher sensitivity of MRI over CT is mostly due to the T2-weighted images. The superior sensitivity of T2-weighted imaging could be explained by an increase in contrast between the coagulated area, which has low signal intensity, and the viable residual tumor, which has high signal intensity. Moreover, the moderately hyperintense area on T2-weighted images associated with corresponding enhancement on contrast-enhanced T1-weighted images offers optimal specificity for residual tumor and recurrent tumor after RFA treatment [34].

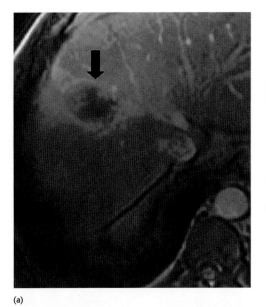

(a)

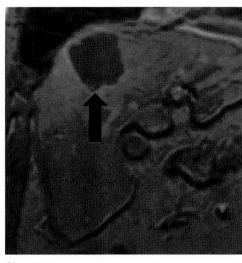

(b)

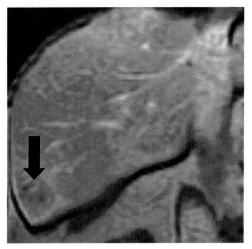

(c)

Figure 3.15 Recurrent tumor seen on MRI 1 month after RFA in a 64-year-old man with a solitary hepatic metastasis from cholangiocarcinoma.
(a) Contrast-enhanced axial T1-weighted imaging in the portal venous phase obtained prior to RFA shows a lesion in segment VIII with irregular enhancement, consistent with metastasis. (b) Contrast-enhanced coronal T1-weighted image obtained 1 month following RFA shows no contrast enhancement within the ablated area (arrow), indicating successful treatment. (c) Contrast-enhanced coronal T1-weighted image of the same patient also shows a new lesion with irregular enhancement in segment VI (arrow), consistent with new metastasis.

Role of PET and PET/CT after RFA

Early recognition of incomplete treatment is therefore a key point for a precise evaluation of the real local efficacy of the RF technology, as well as to ensure optimal long-term outcome [43]. Blokhuis *et al.* [44] reported that the use of PET in combination with CT scan at the follow-up of hepatic malignancies treated with

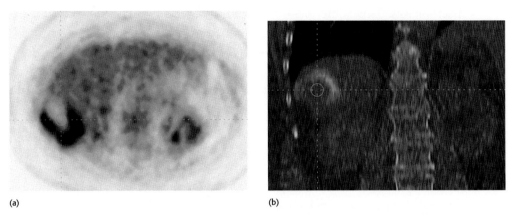

(a)   (b)

Figure 3.16 Recurrent tumor in the 3-month follow-up positron emission tomography/computed tomography (PET/CT) in a 56-year-old woman with a hepatic metastasis from rectal adenocarcinoma after RFA treatment. (a) Axial image shows a rim hypermetabolic area outside the prior treated area over segment IV, consistent with recurrence. (b) Coronal image also demonstrates a rim hypermetabolic area outside the prior treated area over segment IV, consistent with recurrence. *See color plate section.*

RFA might lead to earlier detection (mean period 6.8 months) of tumor recurrence than contrast-enhanced CT alone (mean period 9.8 months). These results are similar to the observation made by Donckier *et al.* [45], who reported that FDG-PET accurately monitors the local efficacy of RFA for treatment of liver metastases, as it recognizes incomplete tumor ablation (four patients at 1 week and 1 month after RFA), not detectable on CT.

On PET/CT, incomplete treatment is defined by the persistence of a hypermetabolic nodule within the treated region when the tumor was hypermetabolic before RFA. A recurrent tumor is defined as the reappearance of a hypermetabolic nodule outside the treated area after a negative first postoperative examination [45,46] (Fig. 3.16). Langenhoff *et al.* [47] reported that the positive predictive value for a positive FDG-PET scan for the detection of local recurrence in liver metastases treated with RFA was 80% and the negative predictive value was 100%. Veit *et al.* [46] also reported that the overall sensitivity for detection of residual tumor is 65% for PET and PET/CT and 44% for CT alone.

Currently, the primary indication for PET/CT is to exclude the presence of extrahepatic metastases or to evaluate equivocal or negative findings on MRI or CT [43]. Because it images the entire body, PET/CT can detect extrahepatic metastases elsewhere in the body, offering a further advantage over MRI or CT [43]. Since FDG is not a tumor-specific substance, an inflammatory process can also accumulate the tracer due to increased metabolic activity of leucocytes and macrophages. This is the major well-known source of false-positive results [47]. Another limitation of FDG-PET is the limited spatial resolution, which may lead to dramatically decreased sensitivity of FDG-PET in lesions less than 1 cm (as low as 21%) [46,48]. False-negative results may also occur when a rim-like tracer distribution at the ablative margin due to tissue regeneration may superimpose on small recurrent foci [46].

Complications

RFA is relatively safe, and complications are rarely reported. The most common complications encountered during radiofrequency ablation of liver tumors are hepatic abscess, intraperitoneal hemorrhage, biloma, ground pad burn, pneumothorax (Fig. 3.17), and vasovagal reflex [49]. Other complications include biliary stricture, diaphragmatic injury, gastric ulcer, hemothorax, hepatic failure, hepatic infarction, renal infarction, sepsis, and transient ischemic attack [49].

Abscess is the most common major complication associated with RFA, and the diagnosis can be sometimes delayed and confused with post-ablation syndrome, which can also present with fever [49]. The imaging features are similar to those of usual hepatic abscess. However, in the presence of air within the lesion, the findings overlap with the microbubbles that can be a common occurrence in a non-infected

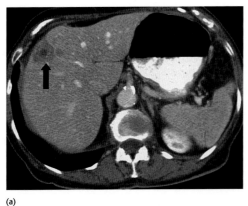
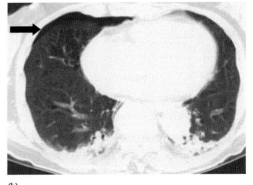

(a)   (b)

Figure 3.17 Pneumothorax following RFA treatment in a 50-year-old man with a solitary hepatic metastasis. (a) Axial CECT image in the portal-venous phase image shows a heterogeneously enhancing metastasis in segment IV. (b) CT image obtained immediately following RFA treatment shows small-volume pneumothorax (arrow) in the right hemithorax. This complication resolved with observation alone.

ablated tumor [49]. Hence, close clinical follow-up is necessary to confirm the diagnosis of abscess. Vascular complications like bleeding, arteriovenous fistula, pseudoaneurysm formation, and hepatic or portal venous thrombosis are not uncommonly encountered, and can be the cause of significant post-procedural morbidity. Prevention, early detection, and proper management are essential for adequate management of these patients [49].

Conclusions

Radiofrequency ablation (RFA) is frequently used to treat hepatocellular carcinoma (HCC) and hepatic metastases, owing to its minimally invasive nature for patients who are not candidates for surgery. Imaging has a central role to play not only in treatment planning prior to RFA, but also in evaluating treatment efficacy after RFA. The advantages and disadvantages of the imaging modalities before and after liver ablation are summarized in Tables 3.6 and 3.7. We predict that RFA will become more and more important and popular in the management of patients with

Table 3.6 Comparison of imaging modalities prior to liver ablation

Parameter	CEUS	MDCT	MRI	PET/CT
Cost	Cheaper	Cheaper	Expensive	Expensive
Reproducibility	Yes	No	No	No
Operator-dependence	Yes	No	No	No
Whole-body survey	No	No	No	Yes
Specificity for lesion characterization	High	High	High	Low
Sensitivity for lesion detection	Low	High	High	High
Radiation	No	Yes	No	Yes

Table 3.7 Comparison of imaging modalities after liver ablation

Parameter	MDCT	MRI	PET/CT
Cost	Cheaper	Expensive	Expensive
Whole-body survey	No	No	Yes
Specificity for detecting residual tumor	High	High	High
Sensitivity for detecting residual tumor	Low	High	High
Radiation	Yes	No	Yes

hepatic malignancies. To achieve better outcome for the patients, it is imperative that clinical operators are familiar with the utility and limitations of the various imaging modalities involved with radiofrequency ablation.

REFERENCES

1. Fong Y, Sun RL, Jarnagin W, Blumgart LH. An analysis of 412 cases of hepatocellular carcinoma at a Western center. *Ann Surg* 1999; **229**: 790–800.
2. Fong Y, Kemeny N, Paty P, Blumgart LH, Cohen AM. Treatment of colorectal cancer: hepatic metastasis. *Semin Surg Oncol* 1996; **12**: 219–52.
3. Hong SN, Lee SY, Choi MS, *et al.* Comparing the outcomes of radiofrequency ablation and surgery in patients with a single small hepatocellular carcinoma and well-preserved hepatic function. *J Clin Gastroenterol* 2005; **39**: 247–52.
4. Vivarelli M, Guglielmi A, Ruzzenente A, *et al.* Surgical resection versus percutaneous radiofrequency ablation in the treatment of hepatocellular carcinoma on cirrhotic liver. *Ann Surg* 2004; **240**: 102–7.
5. Poon RT, Fan ST, Lo CM, Liu CL, Wong J. Intrahepatic recurrence after curative resection of hepatocellular carcinoma: long-term results of treatment and prognostic factors. *Ann Surg* 1999; **229**: 216–22.
6. Pawlik TM, Choti MA. Surgical therapy for colorectal metastases to the liver. *J Gastrointest Surg* 2007; **11**: 1057–77.
7. Gervais DA, Arellano RS, Mueller PR. Percutaneous radiofrequency ablation of ovarian cancer metastasis to the liver: indications, outcomes, and role in patient management. *AJR Am J Roentgenol* 2006; **187**: 746–50.
8. Cho CM, Tak WY, Kweon YO, *et al.* [The comparative results of radiofrequency ablation versus surgical resection for the treatment of hepatocellular carcinoma.] *Korean J Hepatol* 2005; **11**: 59–71.
9. Abdalla EK, Vauthey JN, Ellis LM, *et al.* Recurrence and outcomes following hepatic resection, radiofrequency ablation, and combined resection/ablation for colorectal liver metastases. *Ann Surg* 2004; **239**: 818–27.
10. Goldberg SN, Gazelle GS, Halpern EF, *et al.* Radiofrequency tissue ablation: importance of local temperature along the electrode tip exposure in determining lesion shape and size. *Acad Radiol* 1996; **3**: 212–18.
11. Yu HC, Cheng JS, Lai KH, *et al.* Factors for early tumor recurrence of single small hepatocellular carcinoma after percutaneous radiofrequency ablation therapy. *World J Gastroenterol* 2005; **11**: 1439–44.
12. Harrison LE, Koneru B, Baramipour P, *et al.* Locoregional recurrences are frequent after radiofrequency ablation for hepatocellular carcinoma. *J Am Coll Surg* 2003; **197**: 759–64.

13. Chen MS, Zhang YJ, Li JQ, *et al.* [Randomized clinical trial of percutaneous radiofrequency ablation plus absolute ethanol injection compared with radiofrequency ablation alone for small hepatocellular carcinoma.] *Zhonghua Zhong Liu Za Zhi* 2005; **27**: 623–5.

14. Namasivayam S, Salman K, Mittal PK, Martin D, Small WC. Hypervascular hepatic focal lesions: spectrum of imaging features. *Curr Probl Diagn Radiol* 2007; **36**: 107–23.

15. Sahani DV, Kalva SP. Imaging the liver. *Oncologist* 2004; **9**: 385–97.

16. Brink JA. Use of high concentration contrast media (HCCM): principles and rationale – body CT. *Eur J Radiol* 2003; **45** (Suppl 1): S53–8.

17. Itoh S, Ikeda M, Achiwa M, *et al.* Multiphase contrast-enhanced CT of the liver with a multislice CT scanner: effects of iodine concentration and delivery rate. *Radiat Med* 2005; **23**: 61–9.

18. Awai K, Takada K, Onishi H, Hori S. Aortic and hepatic enhancement and tumor-to-liver contrast: analysis of the effect of different concentrations of contrast material at multi-detector row helical CT. *Radiology* 2002; **224**: 757–63.

19. Wilson SR, Jang HJ, Kim TK, Burns PN. Diagnosis of focal liver masses on ultrasonography: comparison of unenhanced and contrast-enhanced scans. *J Ultrasound Med* 2007; **26**: 775–87.

20. Boozari B, Lotz J, Galanski M, Gebel M. [Diagnostic imaging of liver tumours: current status.] *Internist (Berl)* 2007; **48**: 8–20.

21. Quaia E, Calliada F, Bertolotto M, *et al.* Characterization of focal liver lesions with contrast-specific US modes and a sulfur hexafluoride-filled microbubble contrast agent: diagnostic performance and confidence. *Radiology* 2004; **232**: 420–30.

22. Janica JR, Lebkowska U, Ustymowicz A, *et al.* Contrast-enhanced ultrasonography in diagnosing liver metastases. *Med Sci Monit* 2007; **13** (Suppl 1): 111–15.

23. Braga HJ, Choti MA, Lee VS, *et al.* Liver lesions: manganese-enhanced MR and dual-phase helical CT for preoperative detection and characterization comparison with receiver operating characteristic analysis. *Radiology* 2002; **223**: 525–31.

24. Laghi A. Multidetector CT (64 slices) of the liver: examination techniques. *Eur Radiol* 2007; **17**: 675–83.

25. Schima W, Kulinna C, Langenberger H, Ba-Ssalamah A. Liver metastases of colorectal cancer: US, CT or MR? *Cancer Imaging* 2005; **5** (Spec no A): S149–56.

26. Holalkere NS, Sahani DV, Blake MA, *et al.* Characterization of small liver lesions: added role of MR after MDCT. *J Comput Assist Tomogr* 2006; **30**: 591–6.

27. Lai DT, Fulham M, Stephen MS, *et al.* The role of whole-body positron emission tomography with [18F]fluorodeoxyglucose in identifying operable colorectal cancer metastases to the liver. *Arch Surg* 1996; **131**: 703–7.

28. Desai DC, Zervos EE, Arnold MW, *et al.* Positron emission tomography affects surgical management in recurrent colorectal cancer patients. *Ann Surg Oncol* 2003; **10**: 59–64.

29. Gallowitsch HJ, Kresnik E, Gasser J, *et al.* F-18 fluorodeoxyglucose positron-emission tomography in the diagnosis of tumor recurrence and metastases in the follow-up of patients with breast carcinoma: a comparison to conventional imaging. *Invest Radiol* 2003; **38**: 250–6.

30. Sun L, Wu H, Guan YS. Positron emission tomography/computer tomography: challenge to conventional imaging modalities in evaluating primary and metastatic liver malignancies. *World J Gastroenterol* 2007; **13**: 2775–83.

31. Kula Z, Szefer J, Zuchora Z, Romanowicz G, Pietrzak T. [Evaluation of positron emission tomography by using F-18-fluorodeoxyglucose in diagnosis of recurrent colorectal cancer.] *Pol Merkur Lekarski* 2004; **17** (Suppl 1): 63–6.

32. Goldberg SN, Hahn PF, Tanabe KK, *et al.* Percutaneous radiofrequency tissue ablation: does perfusion-mediated tissue cooling limit coagulation necrosis? *J Vasc Interv Radiol* 1998; **9**: 101–11.

33. Goldberg SN, Solbiati L, Hahn PF, *et al.* Large-volume tissue ablation with radio frequency by using a clustered, internally cooled electrode technique: laboratory and clinical experience in liver metastases. *Radiology* 1998; **209**: 371–9.

34. Dromain C, de Baere T, Elias D, *et al.* Hepatic tumors treated with percutaneous radio-frequency ablation: CT and MR imaging follow-up. *Radiology* 2002; **223**: 255–62.

35. Filippone A, Iezzi R, Di Fabio F, *et al.* Multidetector-row computed tomography of focal liver lesions treated by radiofrequency ablation: spectrum of findings at long-term follow-up. *J Comput Assist Tomogr* 2007; **31**: 42–52.

36. Ninomiya T, Seo Y, Yano Y, *et al.* Evaluation of the therapeutic effect using MD-CT immediately after RFA for HCC. *Hepatogastroenterology* 2006; **53**: 558–60.

37. Nghiem HV, Francis IR, Fontana R, *et al.* Computed tomography appearances of hypervascular hepatic tumors after percutaneous radiofrequency ablation therapy. *Curr Probl Diagn Radiol* 2002; **31**: 105–11.

38. Lim HK, Choi D, Lee WJ, *et al.* Hepatocellular carcinoma treated with percutaneous radio-frequency ablation: evaluation with follow-up multiphase helical CT. *Radiology* 2001; **221**: 447–54.

39. Rossi S, Buscarini E, Garbagnati F, *et al.* Percutaneous treatment of small hepatic tumors by an expandable RF needle electrode. *AJR Am J Roentgenol* 1998; **170**: 1015–22.

40. Goldberg SN, Gazelle GS, Compton CC, Mueller PR, Tanabe KK. Treatment of intrahepatic malignancy with radiofrequency ablation: radiologic–pathologic correlation. *Cancer* 2000; **88**: 2452–63.

41. Rowland IJ, Rivens I, Chen L, *et al.* MRI study of hepatic tumours following high intensity focused ultrasound surgery. *Br J Radiol* 1997; **70**: 144–53.

42. Livraghi T, Goldberg SN, Monti F, *et al.* Saline-enhanced radio-frequency tissue ablation in the treatment of liver metastases. *Radiology* 1997; **202**: 205–10.

43. Anderson GS, Brinkmann F, Soulen MC, Alavi A, Zhuang H. FDG positron emission tomography in the surveillance of hepatic tumors treated with radiofrequency ablation. *Clin Nucl Med* 2003; **28**: 192–7.

44. Blokhuis TJ, van der Schaaf MC, van den Tol MP, *et al.* Results of radio frequency ablation of primary and secondary liver tumors: long-term follow-up with computed tomography and

positron emission tomography-18F-deoxyfluoroglucose scanning. *Scand J Gastroenterol Suppl* 2004; (241): 93–7.

45. Donckier V, Van Laethem JL, Goldman S, *et al.* [F-18] fluorodeoxyglucose positron emission tomography as a tool for early recognition of incomplete tumor destruction after radiofrequency ablation for liver metastases. *J Surg Oncol* 2003; **84**: 215–23.

46. Veit P, Antoch G, Stergar H, *et al.* Detection of residual tumor after radiofrequency ablation of liver metastasis with dual-modality PET/CT: initial results. *Eur Radiol* 2006; **16**: 80–7.

47. Langenhoff BS, Oyen WJ, Jager GJ, *et al.* Efficacy of fluorine-18-deoxyglucose positron emission tomography in detecting tumor recurrence after local ablative therapy for liver metastases: a prospective study. *J Clin Oncol* 2002; **20**: 4453–8.

48. Fong Y, Saldinger PF, Akhurst T, *et al.* Utility of 18F-FDG positron emission tomography scanning on selection of patients for resection of hepatic colorectal metastases. *Am J Surg* 1999; **178**: 282–7.

49. Rhim H, Yoon KH, Lee JM, *et al.* Major complications after radio-frequency thermal ablation of hepatic tumors: spectrum of imaging findings. *Radiographics* 2003; **23**: 123–34.

4

Transarterial chemoembolization in the management of primary and secondary liver tumors

Alexander T. Ruutiainen and Michael Soulen

Introduction

Primary and secondary liver tumors are a common cause of morbidity and mortality around the world. While curative therapies for some of these cancers exist – hepatocellular carcinoma (HCC) can be treated with partial hepatectomy or liver transplantation – many patients are ineligible for curative liver resection due to the advanced stage of their cancers; furthermore, widespread implementation of liver transplantation is prevented by a shortage of donor organs. The same is true for patients with metastatic colorectal or neuroendocrine tumors. Due to these shortcomings, various palliative therapies have been advanced in the management of hepatic neoplasms. These include systemic chemotherapy, radiation therapy, and local and regional percutaneous modalities. The latter group comprises both ablative techniques (chemical and thermal), and the intra-arterial embolotherapies.

Unlike healthy hepatocytes, which are supplied largely by the portal venous circulation, both primary and secondary liver tumors receive their vascular supply principally from the hepatic artery. Thus, occlusion of the hepatic artery would be expected to lead to ischemic necrosis of tumor cells while selectively sparing the native liver. This principle has been exploited in the development of bland transarterial embolization (TAE) and transarterial chemoembolization (TACE). In both of these approaches, the branches of the hepatic artery that supply the tumor are occluded with embolic particles. For chemoembolization, chemotherapeutic agents are added to the embolization mixture for delivery directly into the tumor.

In principle, chemoembolization targets liver lesions by a multifaceted attack. First, embolization of the vascular supply triggers localized tissue ischemia. Second, since the chemotherapeutic agents are delivered directly into the ischemic tumor, their local concentrations and tissue dwell times can be significantly increased [1–5].

Interventional Radiological Treatment of Liver Tumors, ed. Andy Adam and Peter R. Mueller.
Published by Cambridge University Press. © Cambridge University Press 2009.

Equally importantly, the ischemia induced by chemoembolization may counteract drug resistance by causing metabolically active cell membrane pumps to fail, thereby increasing intracellular retention of the chemotherapeutic agents [3,6].

Technique of chemoembolization

Pretreatment assessment

Preoperative evaluation for chemoembolization includes imaging, serology, and counseling. A patient should have either a definitive tissue diagnosis or a compelling clinical diagnosis, such as a markedly elevated serum alpha-fetoprotein (AFP) level associated with an HCC-like mass in a cirrhotic liver [3]. The patient must have a dynamic gadolinium-enhanced MRI or triple-phase CT of the liver. Extrahepatic disease should be excluded by a bone scan and cross-sectional imaging of the chest, abdomen, and pelvis. Serological studies should include CBC, PT, PTT, creatinine, liver function tests, and AFP levels. Due to the demanding nature of this palliative treatment, patients should receive thorough counseling about their regimens. In particular, this discussion should mention the common post-embolization syndrome, the 5–7% risk of serious complications, and the 1–4% chance of periprocedural mortality. The patient and family members should clearly understand that chemoembolization is a palliative regimen with the potential for significant discomfort, risk, and expense.

Embolization procedure

Patients need not be routinely admitted until the morning of their procedure, but they should be advised to fast overnight. On the morning of the procedure, patients are hydrated with 0.9% NSS at $200–300\,\mathrm{cm^3\,h^{-1}}$. Prophylactic medications are administered intravenously, including antibiotics (cefazolin 1 g, metronidazole 500 mg) and antiemetics (odansetron 24 mg, decadron 10 mg, diphenhydramine 50 mg). The evidence for antibiotic prophylaxis is not compelling except for patients without a functioning sphincter of Oddi (e.g., post-Whipple or biliary stent), and not all practitioners administer them routinely.

The patient is sedated, prepped, and draped. Before any embolization is performed, diagnostic angiography of the celiac and superior mesenteric arteries is performed to determine the arterial supply to the liver and to confirm the patency of the portal vein. Because non-target embolization of the gut or gallbladder is a significant cause of morbidity, the origins of the right gastric, supraduodenal, cystic, and other potential extrahepatic arteries must be clearly identified [7].

Once the arterial anatomy has been mapped, a catheter is advanced superselectively into a lobar or segmental branch of the right or left hepatic artery. Typically, the lobe with the greatest tumor burden is embolized first, with subsequent treatments targeting the contralateral side. The chemoembolic mixture is injected into the segmental artery until nearly complete stasis of blood flow is achieved. Intra-arterial lidocaine (30 mg boluses, up to a total of 200 mg) and intravenous fentanyl and midazolam should be used to alleviate discomfort during the procedure.

Post-procedure care

Antibiotics, antiemetics, and intravenous hydration are continued after the embolization (3 L of 0.9% NSS over 24 h). The common post-embolization syndrome must be managed aggressively with palliation of pain, nausea, and fever. Specifically, narcotics, perchlorpromazine, odansetron, decadron, and acetaminophen should be liberally administered. The patient can be discharged with the resumption of oral intake and the cessation of parenteral narcotic therapy. Typically, half of patients are discharged on the first postoperative day, while most of the remainder leave after 2 days [3]. Oral home medications include antibiotics (5 days), antiemetics, and narcotics when needed. Laboratory studies are repeated in 3 weeks to ensure the normalization of liver enzymes. Depending upon the tumor burden and arterial anatomy, a cycle of chemoembolization will include between one and four procedures. Thus, the patient will return for the next embolization in about 4 weeks; treatments alternate between the left and right lobes, as well as any parasitized vessels. Following completion of the treatment cycle, response is assessed with repeat cross-sectional imaging and tumor marker serology. If the response has been inadequate, further rounds of chemoembolization can be administered.

Embolic materials

Choice of embolic particles

Various embolic particles are available on the market. Though they differ in structure, no agent has been conclusively demonstrated to be superior to any other. The first embolic particle to be developed, the gelatin sponge (Gelfoam; Upjohn, Kalamazoo, MI) has been used in the majority (71%) of chemoembolization trials [8]. Historically it has been available in various formulations – particles, cubes, pellet, powder, fragments, and strips – the size of the particles determining how distal the embolization would take place [8]. Notably, use of the powder formulation has been discontinued because of an unfavorable side-effect profile. In all of these formulations, the gelatin causes only temporary devascularization, allowing recanalization to take place in about 2 weeks. A similar temporary occlusion agent has also been developed from cross-linked bovine collagen (Angiostat; Regional Therapeutics, Pacific Palisades, CA).

More permanent embolic particles include polyvinyl alcohol (PVA; several vendors) and trisacryl gelatin spheres (Embosphere microspheres; BioSphere Medical, Rockland, MA). Both of these come in a range of sizes (40–1000 μm), allowing the clinician to select the level of embolization. Less commonly, reports exist of the use of steel coils, starch microspheres, autologous blood clots, and even the herb *Bletilla striata* to embolize the hepatic artery [8]. Recent studies have begun to assess the feasibility of drug-eluting beads, a new approach that may offer an improved pharmacokinetic profile compared to traditional chemoembolization [9].

Choice of chemotherapeutic agents

Several chemotherapeutic agents are available for chemoembolization, for use as monotherapy or in combination. Doxorubicin and cisplatin are the most commonly used single agents [8]. Most reports from Europe and Asia use doxorubicin or epirubicin, whether alone or in combination with mitomycin-C. Centers in the United States prefer cisplatin monotherapy or a combination of 100–150 mg cisplatin, 40–60 mg doxorubicin, and 10–20 mg of mitomycin-C (CAM). Although at least one case series suggested that cisplatin may confer a survival benefit over doxorubicin [10], no randomized trial has shown the superiority of any of these agents [8]. In fact, apparent differences between these agents may be driven by the ability to administer more embolizations in patients treated with cisplatin [10]. In any case, no clear consensus has yet emerged for the superiority of any chemotherapeutic agent or combination.

Choice of emulsion: transarterial oily chemoembolization

The observation that iodized poppyseed oil (Ethiodol; Savage Laboratories, Melville, NY) selectively accumulated in hepatocellular carcinomas led to the incorporation of lipiodol (Guerbet, Aulnay-sous-Bois, France) into chemoembolic regimens. This technique, now known as transarterial oily chemoembolization, has the potential to more accurately target the chemotherapeutic drugs. When iodized oil is injected into the hepatic artery, it travels to the distal arterioles, where it shunts into the terminal portal venules at the pre-sinusoidal level. From there, the oil slowly moves into the sinusoids and becomes trapped in the tumor vessels. In theory, any chemotherapeutic agents suspended in this oily phase would thus be targeted to the liver.

Studies in rabbits [1] and humans [11] have demonstrated that the combination of oily chemoembolization with a particulate agent is superior to oily chemoembolization alone [11]. Such an effect is probably caused by the fact that most chemotherapeutic drugs remain in the aqueous phase of the emulsion. When chemoembolization is performed exclusively with an oily emulsion, continuous arterial inflow elutes out the aqueous drug, even though the oil itself remains suspended in the liver. Particulate-only chemoembolization causes relatively proximal occlusion, allowing continued inflow into the tumor from the portal venules, again diluting the chemotherapeutic drugs and resulting in reduced ischemia. Thus the combination of oil and particles allows the occlusion of both distal arterioles and portal venules – effectively sandwiching the drugs and maintaining tumor ischemia. Additionally, since this technique increases hepatic drug retention, it has the benefit of reduced systemic toxicity.

Efficacy of chemoembolization

Historically, the efficacy of the transarterial embolotherapies has been somewhat controversial. For example, early studies were inconclusive about the efficacy of chemoembolization in the treatment of hepatocellular carcinoma. Nevertheless, evidence has emerged during this decade from several randomized trials that a role exists for chemoembolization in the management of HCC. Though the evidence is slightly less clear for the management of colorectal and neuroendocrine metastases, chemoembolization has nonetheless become established as an important palliative therapy in the oncologist's armamentarium.

Role of chemoembolization in unresectable hepatocellular carcinoma

Initial retrospective cohort studies in the Orient, Europe, and the United States suggested that chemoembolization was effective in the palliation of unresectable

HCC: rates of tumor necrosis ranged from 60% to 100% [3]. Cumulative probability of survival in these studies was 54–88% at one year, 33–64% at 2 years, and 18–51% at 3 years, with the best results obtained by repeated embolizations with a combination of iodized oil, gelfoam, and chemotherapeutic drugs. Survival varied directly with oil uptake and retention, and inversely with tumor volume, stage, and Child class.

Nevertheless, early randomized controlled trials failed to demonstrate a survival benefit for patients with unresectable HCC. Chemoembolization with gelfoam/ doxorubicin ($n = 42$ patients) [12], lipiodol/5-epidoxorubicin ($n = 50$) [13], and gelfoam/lipiodol ($n = 96$) [14] did not increase survival compared to control subjects who received only palliation of pain. Interestingly, however, two of these studies [13,14] did demonstrate non-significant trends towards increased survival from chemoembolization, suggesting that they may have been underpowered to answer this question.

Since that time, however, evidence has begun to mount in favor of chemo-embolization in the management of unresectable HCC. In 2002, two randomized studies demonstrated a clear survival benefit from chemoembolization. In the first study, of 80 patients from Hong Kong, survival in patients treated with cisplatin/ lipiodol/gelatin-sponge chemoembolization was 57%, 31%, and 26% at 1, 2, and 3 years, compared with 32%, 11%, and 3% in those receiving conservative management [15]. In the second study, of 112 patients from Barcelona, 1-year and 2-year survival was 82% and 63% in patients receiving doxorubicin/gelatin-sponge chemoembolization, 75% and 50% in those treated only with gelatin-sponge bland TAE, and 63% and 27% for those receiving conservative management [16]. The authors hypothesized that the results of these trials may have differed from earlier studies because of differences in patient demographics and tumor background [15]. In particular, the studies from Hong Kong and Barcelona were conducted in patients whose HCC arose in the presence of viral hepatitis in 80% of cases, compared to a higher preponderance of alcohol-induced liver disease in the earlier French studies [14]. The tolerance of patients with alcohol-induced cirrhosis for chemoembolization may have been lower than that of those with viral hepatitis [15].

A recent meta-analysis of 175 cohort studies and randomized controlled trials (RCTs) of chemoembolization in the treatment of unresectable HCC concluded that chemoembolization does provide a significant survival benefit when compared to conservative therapy (631 patients in nine RCTs, $p = 0.0025$) [8]. Interestingly, a sub-analysis of studies comparing chemoembolization to bland TAE (412 patients, 3 RCTs) failed to demonstrate a survival benefit for either methodology, though chemoembolization trended towards an improved outcome ($p = 0.052$). Lastly, chronologically later studies demonstrated improved outcomes in comparison to earlier trials [8]; this finding could be partially explained as a result of the improving proficiency of clinicians.

In summary, evidence indicates that patients with unresectable hepatocellular carcinomas benefit from transarterial chemoembolization, though the benefit of specific choices of chemoembolic combinations remains unproven. Disagreements between early randomized trials of chemoembolization and newer studies may have resulted from differences in the patient populations or from the improving proficiency of clinicians.

Role of chemoembolization as a neoadjuvant therapy in HCC

While chemoembolization has become well established as a palliative therapy in the management of unresectable hepatocellular carcinomas, its role as a neoadjuvant therapy for HCC has been more controversial. In theory, chemoembolization could prevent tumor growth in patients awaiting orthotopic liver transplants, thus decreasing attrition from the transplant waiting list due to tumor progression: as such, chemoembolization could serve as a bridge to transplantation. Alternatively, preoperative chemoembolization might be expected to improve outcomes after partial hepatic resection, and might even convert some unresectable lesions into resectable tumors.

Early support for the role of chemoembolization as a neoadjuvant came from retrospective cohort studies showing that neoadjuvant chemoembolization could induce a reduction in tumor size and thus a downstaging of HCC before hepatic resection or liver transplantation [17,18]. Similarly, while the 6-month drop-out rate from the transplant waiting list is typically between 23% and 46% [19], those patients who receive neoadjuvant chemoembolization have been reported to have a drop-out rate of only 15% [20]. Nevertheless, while such early studies were encouraging, it is unclear whether their conclusions can translate to improved outcomes. For example, the aforementioned study [18] failed to demonstrate a statistically significant improvement in patient survival, thus calling into question the clinical relevance of the findings. In fact, the results of later retrospective cohort studies of chemoembolization as a bridge to transplant have been contradictory [19,21], and no RCT has yet been conducted on the issue. In fact, a recent systematic evidence-based review of the available studies concluded that at present there is insufficient evidence to claim that chemoembolization could be used as a bridge to transplant, that it would decrease transplant waiting list drop-out rates, or that preoperative chemoembolization could improve post-transplant survival in patients with HCC [19]. Perhaps the most relevant confounding variable is wait times for listed patients. In regions with short wait times (< 3 months), the drop-out rate is low, so neoadjuvant therapy is not beneficial. When wait times are very long, approaching the median time-to-progression after image-guided therapy, the benefit from neoadjuvant stabilization is lost. The wide geographic and temporal variation in wait times makes analysis of the benefit of neoadjuvant therapy from prior literature difficult. Nevertheless, in the absence of any randomized trials, chemoembolization continues to be used in a non-palliative role in the pre-transplant setting, largely because it at least has not been shown to increase postoperative complications in transplant patients [22].

The effectiveness of preoperative chemoembolization in patients receiving hepatic resection has been similarly controversial. In theory, the combination of chemoembolization with curative surgery might be expected to improve patient outcomes. Moreover, since chemoembolization has been shown to be capable of downstaging tumors [18], it might be able to convert some patients with unresectable lesions into surgical candidates. Indeed, some studies have shown just this, with preoperative chemoembolization significantly improving the 5-year survival of patients undergoing hepatic resection from 19% to 39% [23]. These findings have been further supported by a large retrospective cohort analysis [24]. However, other prospective trials have failed to show a benefit from neoadjuvant chemoembolization before hepatic resection; one prospective study actually demonstrated worsened actuarial survival in chemoembolized patients due to the delay in curative resection [25]. A review of various adjuvant and neoadjuvant therapies in HCC has concluded that there is insufficient evidence to claim that neoadjuvant chemoembolization improves patient survival before resection [26]. Still, in the absence of definitive randomized controlled trials, the issue remains unresolved.

In summary, the role of chemoembolization as a neoadjuvant before liver transplantation or hepatic resection has been rather controversial. Despite positive findings from some studies, the preponderance of evidence has not yet supported such an indication. In fact, where the administration of chemoembolization may delay a definitive therapy, chemoembolization may actually worsen patient survival [25]. Clearly, randomized controlled studies are needed to further clarify these questions.

Role of chemoembolization in colorectal metastases

Hepatic metastases are a common finding in patients with colorectal cancer, appearing in as many as 50% of cases on presentation; moreover, in many patients, the liver is the only site of metastatic involvement. Unfortunately, curative hepatic resection is an option for only about 20% of patients [27]. For the remainder, systemic chemotherapy is the standard of first-line care, with median survivals of 18–20 months using sequential triple-drug regimens.

Numerous case series have demonstrated the feasibility of chemoembolization in treating metastatic colorectal cancer, even among patients who have previously failed systemic chemotherapy. Morphological responses in early studies ranged widely from 25% to 87% [28,29], with median survival varying between 9.3 and 23 months [28,29]. Such results were at least equivalent and probably better than the responses that would have been expected for contemporary systemic chemotherapy in patients who had already failed their initial treatments [29]. Still, such a degree of variation is surprising and may have been attributable to tumor biology [31]: one study later found that the amount of tumor hypervascularity predicted the degree of response to embolization [30].

Only one randomized controlled study has been published comparing the efficacy of chemoembolization against no treatment in the management of colorectal metastases. This British study randomized 61 patients to receive chemoembolization, bland embolization, or no treatment. Though the differences between the arms did not reach statistical significance, the embolization group trended towards improved survival [32]. The greatest effect was noted in the subgroup of patients with less than 50% hepatic replacement. Thus, the field is still awaiting additional prospective studies comparing chemoembolization to conventional treatments in the management of colorectal metastases to the liver. Interestingly, three randomized studies comparing chemoembolization to bland TAE have failed to uncover any differences in efficacy against colorectal metastases [28,32,33]. It remains unclear whether this is due to insufficient power of these studies or to the equivalence between the therapeutic options.

Role of chemoembolization in neuroendocrine tumor metastases

Neuroendocrine tumors comprise a heterogeneous group of cancers arising from the lungs, pancreas, and gastrointestinal tract; they are notable for often secreting biologically active compounds [34]. Though neuroendocrine tumors behave more indolently than adenocarcinomas, they do have malignant potential and frequently metastasize to the liver. When this occurs, the hepatic metastases themselves become the primary determinant of patient morbidity and mortality. Since many patients are not candidates for curative resection, due to their diffuse disease, and because results from systemic chemotherapy for neuroendocrine tumors have been disappointing, a significant role exists for palliative therapies [35].

Recent studies confirm that aggressive management of neuroendocrine metastases – whether by partial hepatic resection, radiofrequency ablation, or chemoembolization – significantly improves patient survival [36]. Controversy remains, however, regarding the best choice among the palliative options. Various small studies have demonstrated symptomatic relief from chemoembolization in 73–100% of patients [34], a biochemical response in 50–91% [34,35], and a morphological response in 50–84% [34]. However, the effect of chemoembolization or bland embolization on the survival of patients with neuroendocrine metastases has never been conclusively established [31]. Moreover, in the past, it has been unclear whether these morphological and symptomatic successes were limited to chemoembolization or could be obtained with bland embolization alone. A retrospective cohort study demonstrated that chemoembolization is superior to bland embolization among the subset of patients with carcinoid neuroendocrine tumors; this benefit was seen without a concomitant increase in toxicity [37]. Nevertheless, future randomized clinical trials are urgently needed to definitively establish any differences in efficacy, and to compare the transarterial treatments to other palliative modalities.

Toxicity of chemoembolization

Despite having a more favorable side-effect profile than conventional chemotherapy, chemoembolization is not free of complications. Thirty-day mortality ranges from 1% to 4%; chemoembolization in the treatment of HCC had a median mortality of 2.4% in a recent meta-analysis of 2858 patients [8]. Severe complications of chemoembolization occur in 5–7% of subjects, though these rates can be reduced to 3–4% when patients are properly selected. Most patients suffer from a self-limited post-embolization syndrome. Major complications of chemoembolization include hepatic insufficiency, abscesses, ischemic complications (cholecystitis, bile duct necrosis, perforation of the alimentary tract), and renal dysfunction. Less commonly, chemoembolization can also lead to tumor rupture, occlusion of the hepatic artery, and clinically significant pancreatitis.

Post-embolization syndrome

The majority of patients (40–86%) [14,38] suffer from a condition termed post-embolization syndrome (PES). This is generally characterized by fever (74% of patients), abdominal pain (45.2%), nausea/emesis (58.9%), and a transaminitis (54%) [39]. In most cases PES is self-limited, though its palliation does necessitate hospitalization. On average, patients defervesce within 3 days, their nausea and pain can be medically managed, and their hepatic function gradually returns to normal [39]. Though previously thought to be indicative of tumor necrosis and thus a successful treatment, neither the presence nor the severity of PES has been shown to correlate to positive patient outcomes [38]. While reliable clinical predictors of the severity of PES have not yet been identified, PES does trend towards a more indolent course when embolization of the gallbladder is avoided, and when the patient is receiving repeat embolization to previously treated territory [7].

Major complications

Acute irreversible hepatic decompensation has been reported to occur in 3% of patients [8,39]. It should be distinguished from the transient and self-limited transaminitis that occurs with post-embolization syndrome. Irreversible decompensation is more common with the use of high doses of cisplatin and poor pretreatment hepatic function (high bilirubin, prolonged PT, and advanced cirrhosis) [39].

Abscess formation affects between 0.2% and 2.5% [40,43] of patients receiving chemoembolization. The majority of these infections occur in the liver, though 0.4% of patients may suffer from a splenic abscess [40]. While their proximate cause is an infectious process, their formation is ultimately permitted by local ischemic necrosis. Abscesses present with localized pain, fever, and leukocytosis, and can be definitively diagnosed by ultrasound or CT [40]. The likelihood of abscess formation has been strongly linked to a history of a Whipple procedure: the presence of a bilioenteric anastomosis increases the incidence of a hepatic abscess by an odds ratio of 894 [41]. Attempts at prophylaxis against the formation of abscesses have led many clinicians to treat patients with broad-spectrum antibiotics peri- and postoperatively [8]; others have even advocated the addition of antibiotics to the embolic mixture. However, a recent prospective cohort study from Germany casts doubt on these practices: patients who did not receive treatment with antibiotics had no more infections or other complications than those who received 3 days of intravenous and 7 days of oral broad-spectrum antibiotics [42].

Severe ischemic complications, other than abscesses, have been reported to occur in 2.1% of patients receiving chemoembolization: these consist of ischemic cholecystitis (1.1%), bile duct necrosis (1.1%) [40], and perforation of the duodenum (0.05%) [43]. However, several other studies have quoted the incidence of gastroduodenal erosions and ulcerations to be significantly higher: one retrospective analysis of 280 cases demonstrated an endoscopy-proven incidence of 5.3% [44]. Since such lesions can result from the reflux of embolic material into the gastric circulation, the importance of meticulous attention to anatomic variants and adherence to selective or superselective embolization is the primary safeguard against this possibility [44]. Alternatively, at least some of these lesions could be the result of stress ulceration. Similarly, embolization distal to the cystic artery is the primary way of avoiding ischemic cholecystitis [40]. Nevertheless, since chemoembolization purposefully causes tissue ischemia, some damage to structures that are dependent on the hepatic artery is unavoidable (e.g., the intrahepatic bile ducts).

Renal failure has also been documented as a complication of chemoembolization, though its reported incidence varies between 0.05% [43] and 13%, averaging 1.8% in the aforementioned meta-analysis [8]. A prospective cohort study revealed an incidence of 8.6%, with 2.9% developing irreversible renal impairment [45]. Independent risk factors for the development of acute renal failure are the number of chemoembolization sessions, high Child–Pugh class, and a severe course of post-embolization syndrome; irreversible renal dysfunction was predicted only by the presence of diabetes [45]. The proximate causes of such kidney damage may be the use of arterial contrast agents, the nephrotoxicity of the chemotherapeutic drugs, and inflammatory factors released from tumor necrosis [8,45].

The less common complications of chemoembolization include tumor rupture, occlusion of the hepatic artery, and clinically significant pancreatitis. Spontaneous rupture of the treated tumor occurs in 0.15% of patients, most often after the embolization of a large neoplasm [43]. Occlusion of the hepatic artery is a complication of repeated embolizations, occurring in 2% of patients following their second or third round of chemoembolization [43]. Though clinically significant pancreatitis is generally considered a rare complication – Roullet *et al.* report an incidence of 1.7% [46] – subclinical elevations in pancreatic enzymes may occur in as many as 15.2% of patients [47].

Patient selection

The likelihood of suffering severe side effects from chemoembolization is attenuated by both meticulous technique and proper patient selection. In principle, patients must be selected to include only those who will both benefit and tolerate the embolization procedure.

Selecting patients for optimum efficacy

Patients with multiple or unresectable lesions located exclusively or predominantly in the liver are ideal candidates for chemoembolization. Since liver embolization only targets intrahepatic lesions, patients whose hepatic tumor burden is the primary driver of their symptoms and survival are the most likely to benefit from chemoembolization. Nevertheless, the presence of some extrahepatic disease is not an absolute contraindication to chemoembolization; some patients whose metastatic disease is minimal or indolent may still be candidates for this therapy.

Selecting patients for optimum tolerability

The fundamental principle underlying the intra-arterial embolotherapies is the differential blood supply of the hepatic neoplasms (supplied via the hepatic artery) and hepatocytes (supplied via the portal vein). Thus, if the native hepatocytes were to become more dependent on the blood flow from the hepatic artery, embolization of this vessel would be expected to lead to increased side effects. This has in fact been demonstrated. Conditions that predispose the healthy liver to injury by increasing the relative contribution of blood from the arterial circulation include portal vein thrombi and superimposed liver disease. Thus, occlusion of the portal vein is a relative contraindication to chemoembolization, though small case series suggest that patients with significant collateral flow can still be embolized safely [48]. Patients with significant liver disease, such as those of Child–Pugh class C, with tumor replacing > 50% of liver [49], alphafetoprotein > 400 U L^{-1} [49], lactate dehydrogenase > 425 IU L^{-1}, aspartate aminotransferase > 100 IU L^{-1}, or total bilirubin ≥ 2 mg dL^{-1}, are also at increased risk. Severe liver disease, as indicated by hepatic encephalopathy or jaundice, is an absolute contraindication to embolization.

Biliary pathology is another relative contraindication. Biliary obstruction predisposes patients to biliary necrosis even in the absence of hyperbilirubinemia.

As discussed previously, a surgical biliary anastomosis or stent virtually guarantees the development of a hepatic abscess, at least in the absence of prophylactic antibiotics [41]. Last, since the chemoembolization procedure must include angiography, patients with contraindications to this procedure cannot be embolized. All of the contraindications for chemoembolization also apply to bland embolization.

New developments in chemoembolization technology

The latest generation of embolic particles are polyvinyl alcohol polymeric beads specifically designed to load chemotherapeutic drugs and elute them over time into the tumor tissue following embolization. Preclinical bench-top and animal studies have confirmed the ability of these drug-eluting beads to provide enhanced local drug delivery over a prolonged period with minimal systemic exposure [50,51]. Phase I/II clinical trials for hepatoma in Europe and Asia have shown promising 1-year and 2-year survivals in the 85–90% range, but a disturbing incidence of major complications at around 10%, with a surprising frequency of hepatic abscess [52,53]. Randomized trials against conventional oily chemoembolization have not been completed. These beads are available as bland embolics in the USA and can be loaded with one or more drugs, but such off-label use is discouraged until their safety and efficacy is established in clinical trials, particularly given their high cost.

Summary

Transarterial chemoembolization is a powerful and well-established tool in the palliative management of both primary and secondary liver tumors. While future randomized trials are still needed to unequivocally prove the survival benefits of chemoembolization in some cancers, its effects on the management of symptoms have been clearly demonstrated. When performed with meticulous technique, chemoembolization can be efficacious while still maintaining a side-effect profile superior to that of conventional therapies. Though patient selection remains crucial, the transarterial embolotherapies can be offered to many more patients than traditional hepatic resection or transplantation. Therefore, familiarity with chemoembolization is essential for any clinician involved in the care of patients with primary or secondary liver tumors.

REFERENCES

1. Konno T. Targeting cancer chemotherapeutic agents by use of lipiodol contrast medium. *Cancer* 1990; **66**: 1897–903.

2. Egawa H, Maki A, Mori K, *et al.* Effects of intraarterial chemotherapy with a new lipophilic anticancer agent, estradiol-chlorambucil (KM2210), dissolved in lipiodol on experimental liver tumor in rats. *J Surg Oncol* 1990; **44**: 109–14.

3. Ramsey DE, Kernagis LY, Soulen MC, Geschwind JF. Chemoembolization of hepatocellular carcinoma. *J Vasc Interv Radiol* 2002; **13**: S211–21.

4. Nakamura H, Hashimoto T, Oi H, Sawada S. Transcatheter oily chemoembolization of hepatocellular carcinoma. *Radiology* 1989; **170**: 783–6.

5. Sasaki Y, Imaoka S, Kasugai H, *et al.* A new approach to chemoembolization therapy for hepatoma using ethiodized oil, cisplatin, and gelatin sponge. *Cancer* 1987; **60**: 1194–203.

6. Kruskal JB, Hlatky L, Hahnfeldt P, *et al.* In-vivo and in-vitro analysis of the effectiveness of doxorubicin combined with temporary arterial occlusion in liver tumors. *J Vasc Interv Radiol* 1993; **4**: 741–8.

7. Leung DA, Goin JE, Sickles C, Soulen MC. Determinants of post-embolization syndrome following hepatic chemoembolization. *J Vasc Interv Radiol* 2001; **12**: 321–6.

8. Marelli L, Stigliano R, Triantos C, *et al.* Transarterial therapy for hepatocellular carcinoma: which technique is more effective? A systematic review of cohort and randomized studies. *Cardiovasc Intervent Radiol* 2007; **30**: 6–25.

9. Varela M, Real MI, Burrel M, *et al.* Chemoembolization of hepatocellular carcinoma with drug eluting beads: efficacy and doxorubicin pharmacokinetics. *J Hepatol* 2007; **46**: 474–81.

10. Ono Y, Yoshimasu T, Ashikaga R, *et al.* Long-term results of lipiodol-transcatheter arterial embolization with cisplatin or doxorubicin for unresectable hepatocellular carcinoma. *Am J Clin Oncol* 2000; **23**: 564–8.

11. Takayasu K, Shima Y, Muramatsu Y, *et al.* Hepatocellular carcinoma: treatment with intraarterial iodized oil with and without chemotherapeutic agents. *Radiology* 1987; **163**: 345–51.

12. Pelletier G, Roche A, Ink O, *et al.* A randomized trial of hepatic arterial chemoembolization in patients with unresectable hepatocellular carcinoma. *J Hepatol* 1990; **1**: 181–4.

13. Madden MV, Krige JE, Bailey S, *et al.* Randomised trial of targeted chemotherapy with lipiodol and 5-epidoxorubicin compared with symptomatic treatment for hepatoma. *Gut* 1993; **34**: 1598–600.

14. Group d'Etude et de Traitement du Carcinome Hépatocellulaire. A comparison of lipiodol chemoembolization and conservative treatment for unresectable hepatocellular carcinoma. *N Engl J Med* 1995; **332**: 1256–61.

15. Lo CM, Ngan H, Tso WK, *et al.* Randomized controlled trial of transarterial lipiodol chemoembolization for unresectable hepatocellular carcinoma. *Hepatology* 2002; **35**: 1164–71.

16. Llovet JM, Real MI, Montana X, *et al.* Arterial embolization or chemoembolization versus symptomatic treatment in patients with unresectable hepatocellular carcinoma: a randomized controlled trial. *Lancet* 2002; **359**: 1734–9.

17. Harada T, Matsuo K, Inoue T, *et al.* Is preoperative hepatic arterial chemoembolization safe and effective for hepatocellular carcinoma? *Ann Surg* 1996; **224**: 4–9.

18. Majno PE, Adam R, Bismuth H, *et al.* Influence of preoperative transarterial lipiodol chemoembolization on resection and transplantation for hepatocellular carcinoma in patients with cirrhosis. *Ann Surg* 1997; **226**: 688–701.

19. Lesurtel M, Müllhaupt B, Pestalozzi BC, Pfammatter T, Clavien PA. Transarterial chemoembolization as a bridge to liver transplantation for hepatocellular carcinoma: an evidence-based analysis. *Am J Transplant* 2006; **6**: 2644–50.

20. Maddala YK, Stadheim L, Andrews JC, *et al.* Drop-out rates of patients with hepatocellular cancer listed for liver transplantation: outcome with chemoembolization. *Liver Transpl* 2004; **10**: 449–55.

21. Oldhafer KJ, Chavan A, Frühauf NR, *et al.* Arterial chemoembolization before liver transplantation in patients with hepatocellular carcinoma: marked tumor necrosis, but no survival benefit? *J Hepatol* 1998; **29**: 953–9.

22. Richard HM 3rd, Silberzweig JE, Mitty HA, *et al.* Hepatic arterial complications in liver transplant recipients treated with pretransplantation chemoembolization for hepatocellular carcinoma. *Radiology* 2000; **214**: 775–9.

23. Di Carlo V, Ferrari G, Castoldi R, *et al.* Pre-operative chemoembolization of hepatocellular carcinoma in cirrhotic patients. *Hepatogastroenterology* 1998; **45**: 1950–4.

24. Zhang Z, Liu Q, He J, *et al.* The effect of preoperative transcatheter hepatic arterial chemoembolization on disease-free survival after hepatectomy for hepatocellular carcinoma. *Cancer* 2000; **89**: 2606–12.

25. Wu CC, Ho YZ, Ho WL, *et al.* Preoperative transcatheter arterial chemoembolization for resectable large hepatocellular carcinoma: a reappraisal. *Br J Surg* 1995; **82**: 122–6.

26. Schwartz JD, Schwartz M, Mandeli J, Sung M. Neoadjuvant and adjuvant therapy for resectable hepatocellular carcinoma: review of the randomised clinical trials. *Lancet Oncol* 2002; **3**: 593–603.

27. Vogl TJ, Zangos S, Eichler K, Yakoub D, Nabil M. Colorectal liver metastases: regional chemotherapy via transarterial chemoembolization (TACE) and hepatic chemoperfusion: an update. *Eur Radiol* 2007; **17**: 1025–34.

28. Martinelli DJ, Wadler S, Bakal CW, *et al.* Utility of embolization or chemoembolization as second-line treatment in patients with advanced or recurrent colorectal carcinoma. *Cancer* 1994; **74**: 1706–12.

29. Lang EK, Brown CL. Colorectal metastases to the liver: selective chemoembolization. *Radiology* 1993; **189**: 417–22.

30. Taniai N, Onda M, Tajiri T, *et al.* Good embolization response for colorectal liver metastases with hypervascularity. *Hepatogastroenterology* 2002; **49**: 1531–4.

31. Goode JA, Matson MB. Embolisation of cancer: what is the evidence? *Cancer Imaging* 2004; **4**: 133–41.

32. Hunt TM, Flowerdew AD, Birch SJ, *et al.* Prospective randomised trial of hepatic arterial embolization or infusion chemotherapy with 5-fluorouracil and degradable starch microspheres for colorectal liver metastases. *Br J Surg* 1990; **77**: 779–82.

33. Salman HS, Cynamon J, Jagust M, *et al*. Randomized phase II trial of embolization therapy versus chemoembolization therapy in previously treated patients with colorectal carcinoma metastatic to the liver. *Clin Colorectal Cancer* 2002; **2**: 173–9.

34. Kaltsas GA, Besser GM, Grossman AB. The diagnosis and medical management of advanced neuroendocrine tumors. *Endocr Rev* 2004; **25**: 458–511.

35. Ruszniewski P, O'Toole D. Ablative therapies for liver metastases of gastroenteropancreatic endocrine tumors. *Neuroendocrinology* 2004; **80** (Suppl 1): 74–8.

36. Touzios JG, Kiely JM, Pitt SC, *et al*. Neuroendocrine hepatic metastases: does aggressive management improve survival? *Ann Surg* 2005; **241**: 776–83.

37. Ruutiainen AT, Soulen MC, Tuite CM, *et al*. Chemoembolization and bland embolization of neuroendocrine tumor metastases to the liver. *J Vasc Interv Radiol* 2007; **18**: 847–55.

38. Wigmore SJ, Redhead DN, Thomson BN, *et al*. Postchemoembolisation syndrome: tumour necrosis or hepatocyte injury? *Br J Cancer* 2003; **89**: 1423–7.

39. Chan AO, Yuen MF, Hui CK, Tso WK, Lai CL. A prospective study regarding the complications of transcatheter intraarterial lipiodol chemoembolization in patients with hepatocellular carcinoma. *Cancer* 2001; **94**: 1747–52.

40. Tarazov PG, Polysalov VN, Prozorovskij KV, Grishchenkova IV, Rozengauz EV. Ischemic complications of transcatheter arterial chemoembolization in liver malignancies. *Acta Radiol* 2000; **41**: 156–60.

41. Kim W, Clark TW, Baum RA, Soulen MC. Risk factors for liver abscess formation after hepatic chemoembolization. *J Vasc Interv Radiol* 2001; **12**: 965–8.

42. Plentz RR, Lankisch TO, Basturk M, *et al*. Prospective analysis of German patients with hepatocellular carcinoma undergoing transcatheter arterial chemoembolization with or without prophylactic antibiotic therapy. *J Gastroenterol Hepatol* 2005; **20**: 1134–6.

43. Xia J, Ren Z, Ye S, *et al*. Study of severe and rare complications of transarterial chemoembolization (TACE) for liver cancer. *Eur J Radiol* 2006; **59**: 407–12.

44. Leung TK, Lee CM, Chen HC. Anatomic and technical skill factor of gastroduodenal complication in post-transarterial embolization for hepatocellular carcinoma: a retrospective cohort study of 280 cases. *World J Gastroenterol* 2005; **11**: 1554–7.

45. Huo TI, Wu JC, Lee PC, Chang FY, Lee SD. Incidence and risk factors for acute renal failure in patients with hepatocellular carcinoma undergoing transarterial chemoembolization: a prospective study. *Liver Int* 2004; **24**: 210–15.

46. Roullet MH, Denys A, Sauvanet A, *et al*. [Acute clinical pancreatitis following selective transcatheter arterial chemoembolization of hepatocellular carcinoma.] *Ann Chir* 1995; **127**: 779–82.

47. Lopez-Benitez R, Radeleff BA, Barragan-Campos HM, *et al*. Acute pancreatitis after embolization of liver tumors: frequency and associated risk factors. *Pancreatology* 2007; **7**: 53–62.

48. Pentecost MJ, Daniels JR, Teitelbaum GP, Stanley P. Hepatic chemoembolization: safety with portal vein thrombosis. *J Vasc Intervent Radiol* 1993; **4**: 347–51.

49. Llado L, Virgili J, Figueras J, *et al*. A prognostic index of survival of patients with unresectable hepatocellular carcinoma after transcatheter arterial chemoembolization. *Cancer* 2000; **88**: 50–7.

50. Lewis AL, Gonzalez MV, Lloyd AW, *et al.* DC Bead: in vitro characterization of a drug-delivery device for transarterial chemoembolization. *J Vasc Intervent Radiol* 2006; **17**: 335–42.

51. Hong K, Khwaja A, Liapi E, *et al.* New intra-arterial drug delivery system for the treatment of liver cancer: preclinical assessment in a rabbit model of liver cancer. *Clin Cancer Res* 2006; **12**: 2563–7.

52. Varela M, Real MI, Burrel M, *et al.* Chemoembolization of hepatocellular carcinoma with drug eluting beads: efficacy and doxorubicin pharmacokinetics. *J Hepatol* 2007; **46**: 474–81.

53. Poon RT, Tso WK, Pang RW, *et al.* A phase I/II trial of chemoembolization for hepatocellular carcinoma using a novel intra-arterial drug-eluting bead. *Clin Gastroenterol Hepatol* 2007; **5**: 1100–8.

5

High-intensity focused ultrasound (HIFU) treatment of liver cancer

Gail ter Haar, Sadaf Zahur, and Chaturika Jayadewa

Introduction

In the past, surgery has frequently been the only viable treatment available for solid tumors. Technological advances have, however, led to a shift towards less invasive tumor destruction techniques such as radiotherapy, laparoscopic surgery, and energy-based methods. These include radiofrequency, laser, and cryo-ablation, and HIFU (high-intensity focused ultrasound). There are a number of reasons why non-invasive techniques are appealing: they are usually associated with lower levels of morbidity and mortality, and may often be conducted as day-case procedures under local anesthetic or sedation. In this chapter, the current status of HIFU for the treatment of liver cancer is presented.

Principles of HIFU

Ultrasound is a mechanical form of energy that can propagate through tissue. At the frequencies used in medicine (0.5–20 MHz) the characteristic millimeter wavelengths in tissue mean that it is possible to bring the energy contained in an ultrasound beam to a tight focus a few centimeters from its source. While low-power ultrasound, as used in diagnostic imaging, passes through tissue without causing cellular damage, at high powers the energy concentrated within the focus may be sufficient to lead to cell death, but only within this focal volume, sparing surrounding tissues. This concept is analogous to using a magnifying glass to focus the sun's rays onto tinder with the aim of starting a fire. Combustion is only achieved when the tight focal spot coincides with the dry material.

Figure 5.1 shows a HIFU lesion. This is the term used to describe the ellipsoidal region of damage whose long axis lies along the direction of propagation of the

Interventional Radiological Treatment of Liver Tumors, ed. Andy Adam and Peter R. Mueller.
Published by Cambridge University Press. © Cambridge University Press 2009.

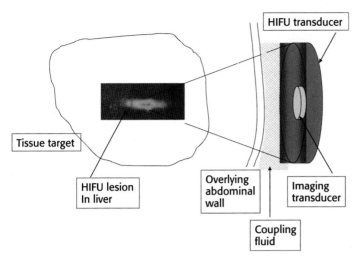

Figure 5.1 Schematic diagram showing the principle of ultrasound-guided extra-corporeal high-intensity focused ultrasound (HIFU). A single HIFU lesion is shown in a piece of bovine liver. The selective nature of the damage is clear.

ultrasound beam. The selective nature of the cell killing can clearly be seen. There is no damage to the tissue lying between the point of entry of the HIFU beam into tissue and the focus. Histology and electron microscopy have shown that the margin between live and dead cells at the lesion edge may be as narrow as six cells wide [1]. Typically, in abdominal applications of HIFU, these lesions are 1–2 cm long, and 2–3 mm in diameter. They are formed using intensities of ~1500 W cm^{-2}. This should be compared with the intensities of ~0.1 W cm^{-2} used in imaging.

The main mechanism for the biological change produced when high-intensity ultrasound travels through tissue is thermal. It is known from thermal biology studies that protein denaturation occurs when a cell is heated to 56 °C for at least a second, or its thermal equivalent. Broadly, at temperatures over 43 °C, for every degree increase in temperature, the time required to achieve a given level of cellular damage is halved [2,3]. The outer edge of the lesion shown in Figure 5.1, which resulted from a 1-second exposure, therefore corresponds to the 56 °C for 1 second thermal dose contour. Temperatures within the center of the lesion will have been significantly higher than this, probably in excess of 80 °C.

The second mechanism for tissue damage in a HIFU field is acoustic cavitation [4]. Ultrasound propagates through tissue as a pressure wave. During the negative portion of the pressure cycle, gas may be drawn out of intercellular fluids. The bubbles so formed are alternately compressed and expanded under the action of the ultrasonic wave, and gradually grow in size. When they reach a diameter that is resonant for the frequency driving them (~3 μm at 1 MHz) the bubbles can suddenly grow very large, and collapse rapidly. This is known as inertial (or collapse) cavitation. Very high temperatures and shear stresses are generated around the collapsing bubble, leading to highly localized mechanical and thermal damage.

The relevance of gas bubbles to HIFU treatments is twofold. The bubbles formed scatter ultrasound strongly, and the scattered energy is absorbed locally, thus increasing the temperature in their vicinity. Another advantage of the presence of bubbles is that they show up as bright echoes on an ultrasound scan. Since they are only formed where the ultrasound energy is greatest, they can provide a useful means of monitoring tissue effects at the focus [5].

When viewed histologically, tissue within the HIFU focus has the appearance of coagulative necrosis. In addition, where cavitation and/or boiling of tissue water has taken place, there are clear holes (or tears) in the tissue.

The liver is covered with a connective tissue capsule that branches and extends throughout the liver as septae. This connective tissue provides a scaffolding of support and the route through which afferent blood vessels, lymphatic vessels, and bile ducts pass. Additionally, the sheets of connective tissue divide the parenchyma of the liver into smaller structural units called lobules. These roughly hexagonal-shaped lobules consist of hepatocytes radiating outward from a central vein. Portal triads, containing a bile duct and a terminal branch of the hepatic artery and portal vein, are found at the vertices of the lobules. Lobules are particularly easy to see in porcine liver, as in this species they are well delineated by connective tissue septae (Fig. 5.2).

Under low magnification (× 20) the lesion margin appears as a hemorrhagic rim (Fig. 5.3). At higher magnification, several regions can be identified (Fig. 5.4). The central portion shows most damage, and often lacks cellular structure (region 1 on Fig. 5.4). This is surrounded by a layer of cells that is characterized by less intense staining and greater extracellular spacing than seen in normal liver (region 2). These regions are enclosed by the hemorrhagic rim (region 3), the periphery of which shows holes. These holes are roughly spherical and are, on average, less than 10 μm in diameter. The holes extend beyond the hemorrhagic rim to the next distinct border, which consists of cells with condensed nuclei (region 4). The nuclei in this area are much smaller than normal hepatocyte nuclei. It is important to note that this border consists of a mixture of normal-looking hepatocytes and condensed nuclei. Additionally, some nuclei show characteristic apoptotic features such as

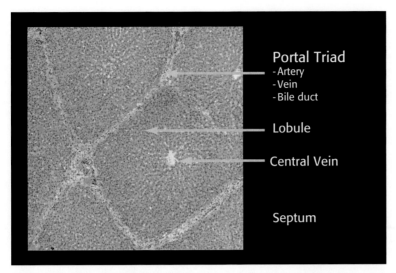

Figure 5.2 Hematoxylin and eosin (H&E) stained section of porcine liver tissue showing normal structure of the liver. *See color plate section*.

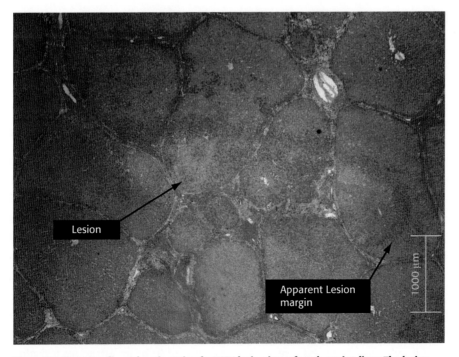

Figure 5.3 Hematoxylin and eosin stain of a HIFU lesion in perfused porcine liver. The lesion is enclosed within the hemorrhagic rim (× 20). *See color plate section*.

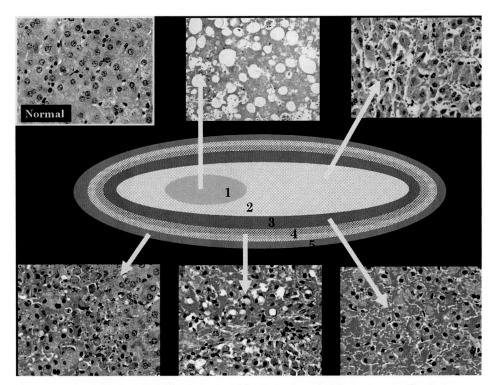

Figure 5.4 Schematic of a HIFU lesion stained with hematoxylin and eosin (× 200 magnification).
The different bands of tissue destruction referred to in the text may be seen. (1) Central region,
showing most distinct damage and regions lacking cellular structure. (2) Region showing less intense
staining, and increased extracellular spacing. (3) Hemorrhagic rim. (4) Region which overlaps regions
3 and 5 and contains "holes." (5) Region in which some hepatocyte nuclei appear condensed.
See color plate section.

nuclear clumping (pyknosis) and granulation (karyolysis). However, it is difficult to determine whether these are apoptotic nuclei or nuclear debris from damaged cells. This border of cells, consisting of condensed nuclei, may represent the true margin of the lesion. Information gathered from hematoxylin and eosin (H&E) stains is, however, insufficient to allow accurate definition of the margin.

The ability of HIFU to target subcutaneous tissue has made it an attractive non-invasive therapy for deep-seated soft-tissue tumors. Malignant cancers of the liver, kidney, breast, and pancreas have been successfully targeted [6–9]. Where bowel gas lies in the propagation path, care must be taken to avoid it. In some treatment orientations it may be successfully displaced using the applied pressure from a water balloon placed against the abdomen. HIFU has proved to be an attractive technique for the treatment of uterine fibroids [10,11]. These may be clearly visualized on magnetic resonance (MR) or ultrasound (US) imaging. While the treatment of benign masses does not necessitate the achievement of confluent tissue ablation, the best prognosis appears to be for those for which the majority of the tumor is targeted [12].

Due to its inability to penetrate gas or bone, at first sight HIFU does not seem to be an appropriate treatment approach for tumors of the lung, bone, or brain. Osteosarcoma has, however, been treated successfully in cases in which it has broken through the bone cortex. Adaptive focusing or "time reversal" techniques are being developed to allow trans-skull treatment of targets in the brain [13–17]. In the absence of such techniques, the ultrasound beam is strongly scattered by the bone, with high absorption of any sound entering the skull. The techniques under investigation, which involve compensating for these effects, result in low intensities at the bone surface (thus reducing potential undesired heating) and re-focusing of the ultrasound beam in the brain. While this technique has mainly been studied with the aim of facilitating non-invasive HIFU treatment of brain tumors, it has application in the liver, where the rib cage presents an obstacle to the HIFU beam. Lung tumors remain difficult to treat because of the air-filled alveoli. However, lung surface tumors may be targeted.

Apart from the prostate, for which specific HIFU treatment devices have been developed [18], the most common clinical usage of HIFU to date has been for tumors of the liver, uterus, kidney, breast, and pancreas [7–9, 19–23]. In the West, these treatments have all been carried out in the context of clinical trials, and the results have been promising. For malignant disease, the organ for which the largest number of treatments has been carried out is the liver.

Treatment devices and procedures

Commercial clinical HIFU devices fall into two broad categories – extracorporeal and transrectal [24]. The most common application of HIFU in oncology, at present, is for the treatment of primary and recurrent prostate cancer. For this, the HIFU transducer is mounted at the end of a transrectal probe, similar in appearance to that used for transrectal ultrasound imaging (TRUS). The aim of these treatments is to destroy the whole gland, since the cancer foci cannot be delineated on an ultrasound image. Abdominal tumor treatments are usually delivered using an extracorporeal HIFU system. In these devices, the transducer is mounted outside the body, and the sound is coupled into the target using a degassed water bath in contact with the skin. Two types of extracorporeal device exist, differing mainly in the mode of imaging used.

Effective HIFU treatments consist of a number of different steps. The initial diagnosis is usually made from a CT or MRI scan. It must then be ascertained whether there is a suitable acoustic window through which the treatment can be delivered, ensuring that the target boundaries can be clearly identified, and that no sensitive normal tissue structures lie in the beam path. The target must then be accurately identified and localized. The next stage in the treatment is to determine the correct ultrasound exposure to achieve ablation. This may be decided in a number of ways. Where ultrasound imaging is used for guidance, the most common method is to use a combination of focal peak intensity and exposure time that results in a hyperechoic region at the target, whereas under MR guidance this combination is varied until the required temperature (and hence thermal dose), as seen using MR thermometry, is reached [25].

During treatment delivery an indicator of tissue effect is needed. This enables assessment of treatment progress, and may also provide feedback to allow adjustment of exposure parameters in real time. This has been done in a number of ways. For MR-guided HIFU, the temperature rise may be determined using spin-lattice relaxation time (T1), proton resonance frequency (PRF), or proton diffusion (D) related sequences. For US-guided treatments, the most commonly used indicator of tissue ablation is the appearance of a hyperechoic region on the image, but other techniques such as elastography and ultrasound thermometry are under active investigation [25].

The final phase of the HIFU procedure is post-treatment assessment of the treatment. Contrast-enhanced MR and ultrasound imaging are used to visualize the vasculature. Successful HIFU ablation leads to occlusion of blood vessels in the target volume, and thus leads to reduced contrast uptake following treatment [26].

Ultrasound is generated from a piezoelectric crystal. In order to produce the focused beams required for HIFU the crystal usually takes the form of a spherical cap. The geometry of the transducer and its resonant frequency determine the shape, size, and position of the focus. If the transducer is formed from a single crystal (element) the focal volume has a fixed shape, whereas if a multi-element phased array is used, the focal geometry and position can be changed electronically. The small size of the focal region means that it is necessary to scan the focus throughout the target volume in an attempt to ablate the whole tumor. This can be achieved by a combination of physical translation of the treatment head and electronic control of the transducer elements. In practice, the target volume is the visible tumor and a normal tissue margin (usually chosen to reflect the surgical resection margin).

The ExAblate (InSightec, Israel) uses MR imaging. The therapeutic ultrasound treatment head comprises a 208-element phased-array transducer with the elements arranged to form the surface of a spherical bowl; it is made of MR-compatible materials and is integrated into the bed of the MR scanner. The HIFU beam is therefore directed upwards, with the patient's skin being coupled to the sound field with aqueous gel spread on the membrane, which seals the water bath that is integral to the scanner bed. The MR scanner not only provides excellent anatomical images, but also offers the possibility of using thermometry sequences to provide thermal dose maps during the course of a HIFU treatment.

The only other widely used extracorporeal clinical system (the Model-JC Tumor Therapy System; Chongqing HAIFU Technology Company, China) relies on US imaging for treatment guidance and monitoring. Again, the transducer sits in a water bath integral to the patient bed, but in this case the US imaging probe is positioned in the center of the therapy treatment head. With this configuration, the imaging and therapy beams remain coaxial, and effectively real-time images are obtained. Ablation in a region is complete when a hyperechoic region is seen on the US image. The thermally ablated region is not visible on standard B-mode images unless gas bubbles have been induced. It is not yet certain whether these are generated by acoustic cavitation or by boiling of the tissue water. Elastographic techniques will eventually allow treatments to be monitored in real time, since the stiffness of tissue is altered by the ablation process [25,27,28]. However, this technique has not yet been adopted clinically. The speed of sound is temperature-dependent, and imaging techniques that make use of this property may be used to locate and place the focus using a low-powered "siting" shot. The apparent change in position of echoes when images of heated and unheated tissues are compared is due to these changes in sound speed. The speed of sound versus temperature curve for soft tissues peaks around 55 °C, and thus this is not a useful technique for detecting threshold ablation temperatures, although a number of researchers are looking for ways around this [25,29].

In both these clinical devices, the treatment head can be moved under computer control, allowing the rotation, tilt, and vertical motion necessary to target the desired volume. While US has the advantage of providing rapid imaging during HIFU exposures, MR is capable of providing images of tissues lying behind bone (including the rib cage) that are not accessible to US imaging beams.

Liver cancer

There are several types of primary liver cell carcinoma, the most common being hepatocellular carcinoma (HCC). HCC is the fifth most common malignancy in the world [30], with 80% of cases developing in cirrhotic livers. HCC is now the leading cause of death among cirrhosis patients in Europe [31].

Hepatitis B virus (HBV) is the most frequent underlying cause of HCC, since it accounts for some 85% of cases in eastern and southeastern Asia and sub-Saharan Africa, where the virus is endemic. Between 70% and 90% of HBV-related HCC develops in patients with cirrhosis. Other risk factors for HCC include hepatitis C virus (HCV), particularly in the West and Japan (32), alcohol abuse (which can act synergistically with HCV to promote carcinogenesis), cirrhosis from any origin, inherited metabolic disorders such as hemochromatosis and tyrosinemia, and dietary aflatoxin exposure. Men are 2 to 4 times more frequently affected by HCC than are women [33].

There are three basic types of HCC: nodular, massive, and diffuse infiltrative [34,35]. The nodular form is the most common, showing distinct solitary or multiple nodules of various sizes and distributions, with the largest focus of tumor presumed to be the primary site. The nodules appear as foci of soft, yellow-green material often with central necrosis. The massive type forms a large discrete mass that replaces all or most of one lobe, with small intrahepatic metastases being detectable in the remainder of the hepatic parenchyma. Diffuse infiltrative HCC is invariably associated with cirrhosis, and shows numerous small nodules of tumor scattered throughout the liver. These are often difficult to distinguish from cirrhotic nodules. All three types may produce liver enlargement, but this is particularly true for the nodular and massive types. Tumor is more often found in the right lobe than in the left, probably because of its greater bulk, and is commonly accompanied with a degree of necrosis and hemorrhage. Infiltration of the diaphragm is common, and the invasion of venous vasculature is a striking feature.

The natural history of the HCC depends on the severity of the underlying cirrhosis, tumor characteristics (size, presence or absence of vascular invasion, pathological grade, and extrahepatic metastases), performance status of the patient, comorbid conditions, and the efficacy of treatment interventions. Several staging systems have been developed, although none is perfect. The Okuda classification uses a gross assessment of tumor factors and is not very useful in the clinical evaluation of patients. The Barcelona Clinic Liver Cancer (BCLC), the Cancer of the Liver Italian Program (CLIP), and the Groupe d'Etude et de Traitement du Carcinome Hépatocellulaire (GETCHC) classifications use more refined assessments. The European and American scientific societies have agreed the common use of the BCLC classification, which links tumor stage with treatment strategy (Table 5.1).

Table 5.1 Barcelona Clinic Liver Cancer Staging Classification of patients with hepatocellular carcinoma [36]

Staging	Performance status	Tumor stage	Child–Pugh
(A) Early	0	Single < 5 cm, 3 nodes < 3 cm	A and B
(B) Intermediate	0	Large/multinodular	A and B
(C) Advanced	1–2	Vascular invasion extrahepatic spread	A and B
(D) End-stage	3–4	Any of the above	C

Metastatic involvement of the liver is far more common than primary liver carcinoma. Although the most common primary sites giving rise to liver metastases are breast, lung, and colon, tumors from any site of the body can spread to the liver, as may lymphomas and leukemias. Typical gross appearance is of multiple nodular metastases which are firm and white, cause striking enlargement of the liver, and may replace up to 80% of normal liver tissue. There is a tendency for metastatic deposits to outgrow their blood supply, thus producing central necrosis and umbilication when viewed from the surface.

HIFU in the treatment of liver tumors

HIFU remains the only minimally invasive extracorporeal ablative technique used for the treatment of liver tumors. HIFU has been administered in the trial setting at centers in China and the UK. Wu *et al.* [22] conducted a prospective non-randomized clinical trial of 55 patients with HCC and cirrhosis to assess safety and efficacy of the treatment. Of these, 51 had unresectable HCC, with tumor size ranging from 4 to 14 cm in diameter with a mean diameter of 8.14 cm. All patients were staged using the tumor, nodes, metastasis (TNM) classification. Fifteen patients corresponded to stage II, 16 to stage IIIA, and 24 to stage IIIC. All patients had HIFU treatment, with the median number of sessions being 1.69. No serious adverse events were reported; complications and side effects were reported in 13 patients. Two patients had low-grade fever up to 38.5 °C, which had resolved 5 days after treatment. Six patients had superficial burns and four had transient pain, with one requiring a prescription for oral analgesia. Follow-up imaging showed an absence of tumor vascular supply and the shrinkage of treated lesions. Serum tumor marker AFP returned to normal in 34% of patients and overall survival rates at 6, 12, and 18 months were 86.1%, 61.5%, and 35.3%, respectively.

The same clinical investigators evaluated the role of combining liver HIFU with transarterial chemoembolization (TACE) for the treatment of advanced hepatocellular carcinoma [23]. Over a 2-year period, 50 patients with advanced hepatocellular carcinoma were enrolled onto one of two treatment groups: TACE performed alone (26 patients) or TACE with HIFU 2–4 weeks later (24 patients). Tumor size ranged from 4 to 14 cm diameter, and all patients were followed for a mean of 8 months (range 3–24 months). Median survival time was found to be 11.3 months in the TACE-with-HIFU group, compared to 4 months in the TACE-only group. The 6-month survival rate was 80.4–85.4% in the TACE-with-HIFU group, compared to 13.2% in the TACE-only group. The 1-year survival rate was 42.9% and 0%, respectively. Similarly, tumor size reduction was much more marked in the TACE-with-HIFU group.

HIFU ablation is also being used in the palliative setting to treat those with advanced liver carcinoma. Li *et al.* [37] reported on 100 patients with liver cancer who underwent HIFU treatment, 62 being primary cases and 38 metastatic cases. After treatment, clinical symptom relief was found in 86.6% of patients; ascites disappeared in six patients and serum tumor markers were lowered by greater than 50% in 65.3% of those with primary liver cancer. Follow-up imaging confirmed coagulative necrosis and blood-supply reduction or tumor disappearance in the target region.

In Oxford, UK, Illing *et al.* [6] performed a prospective, non-randomized clinical trial on 22 patients with metastatic liver carcinoma and 8 patients with kidney cancer. Each liver cancer patient had one or more solid tumor deposits within the organ. Fifteen of the 22 liver cases were non-surgical candidates, and the remaining 7 had surgical resection of their tumor within 14 days of the HIFU treatment. Previous surgery, chemotherapy, or biological therapies were permitted provided the patients had recovered from any related side effects, but no patients had received radiotherapy to the target region. Patients were required to have normal bone function, renal function, coagulation profile, and adequate hepatic reserve. Each patient received contrast-enhanced MRI, baseline blood tests, and symptom review prior to HIFU treatment. A single HIFU treatment session was given under general anesthetic. Radiological follow-up was at day 12, with repeat blood analyses and symptom reviews at days 1, 2, and 12. Primary end points were adverse events and variations in clinical laboratory data during the first 28 days following treatment or until surgical resection, and secondary end points were radiological and histological assessment of response. Evidence of ablation was seen in 93% of patients. MRI assessment showed that the HIFU lesions were placed directly in the tumor in 88% of cases, and for the remainder the ablated region lay within 5 mm of the target. The median area of ablation seen on MRI was 45% smaller than that predicted at the time of treatment, but the histological zones of ablation correlated more closely, with a median area of ablation of 102% of the intended area.

All adverse events of therapy were local to the treatment site and self-limiting. Eighty percent of cases reported discomfort, although this was generally mild in severity. Skin toxicity was seen in eight cases, seven being pinhead blisters which resolved spontaneously and one being grade 2 toxicity, which also resolved spontaneously. Subcutaneous edema which resolved spontaneously was seen in eight patients. Low-grade fever and general malaise was experienced by 13% of patients. This occurred within the first 12 hours and settled within 24 hours. Other literature-reported complications of HIFU treatment, such as damage to bowel or secondary infection of the necrotic tissue, was not observed. Laboratory data showed stability of hepatic function, although a transient elevation in inflammatory markers consistent with a physiological response to tumor ablation was seen. This was not clinically significant.

The Oxford team identified potential limitations to the clinical application of HIFU, which included planning and delivery of treatment. Tumors in the dome of the liver are not likely to be suitable for treatment, because of the proximity of air-filled bowel and lung, through which HIFU beams cannot be directed, or the presence of bone, which can absorb or reflect the ultrasound beam. Treatments of tumors positioned close to bowel or the gallbladder have an increased risk of visceral perforation if the patient should move during the treatment. With the system used by the Oxford team, even without such complicating factors, tumors at depths greater than 10 cm from the skin were less likely to be ablated successfully due to the attenuation of the HIFU energy by normal tissues in the beam path. The treatment time for HIFU is longer than desirable, being up to 2 hours for a 2–3 cm superficially lying tumor; this may make HIFU less favorable than other minimally invasive treatment modalities such as radiofrequency ablation (RFA). However, treatment time is likely to reduce as experience is gained, improvements in technology occur, and combinations with other modalities (such as TACE, discussed above) are investigated.

Another concern has been the possibility that HIFU may promote the spread of metastases. Early studies by Fry and Johnson [38] showed enhancement of metastases after ablation, but recent experimental studies have not confirmed this. On the contrary, a lower metastatic rate in animals treated with HIFU as compared with the control group was observed [39–42]. Wu et al. [43] conducted a study using gene testing on 26 patients, of whom 10 had HCC, and concluded that there was no increased risk of metastases in patients with malignant carcinoma. The same group also conducted a study [44] whose results suggested that HIFU could lead to enhancement of systemic anti-tumor cellular immunity in addition to direct tumor destruction. However, the anti-tumor immune system is very complicated, and it is not known whether the anti-tumor immunity obtained after HIFU treatment is caused by tumor breakdown products or directly by ultrasound ablation.

Summary

HIFU has been demonstrated by the above studies to be a safe, non-invasive treatment option for liver cancer in a range of clinical settings. It is a potentially curative and repeatable treatment. Its benefits include a lower morbidity than more traditional treatment options such as surgery, and its ability to treat a large range of different tumor types. Real-time imaging allows evaluation of the target tissue during treatment, and current imaging modalities can provide accurate therapy outcome measures. HIFU has a potential role in upgrading immunity in the treatment recipient, and no studies have shown a convincing association with an increased risk of metastases.

ACKNOWLEDGEMENT

The authors would like to thank James McLaughlan for providing the lesion photograph in Figure 5.1.

REFERENCES

1. ter Haar GR, Robertson D. Tissue destruction with focused ultrasound in vivo. *Eur Urol* 1993; **23** (Suppl 1): 8–11.
2. Sapareto DG, Dewey WC. Thermal dose determination in cancer therapy. *Br J Radiat Oncol Biol Phys Med* 1984; **10**: 787–800.
3. ter Haar GR, Stratford IJ, Hill CR. Ultrasonic irradiation of mammalian cells in vitro at hyperthermia temperatures. *Br J Radiol* 1980; **53**: 784–9.
4. Coussios CC, Farny CH, ter Haar G, Roy RA. Role of acoustic cavitation in the delivery and monitoring of cancer treatment by high-intensity focused ultrasound (HIFU). *Int J Hyperthermia* 2007; **23**: 105–20.

5. Bailey MR, Couret LN, Sapozhnikov OA, *et al*. Use of overpressure to assess the role of bubbles in focused ultrasound lesion shape in vitro. *Ultrasound Med Biol* 2001; **27**: 695–708.

6. Illing RO, Kennedy JE, Wu F, *et al*. The safety and feasibility of extracorporeal high-intensity focused ultrasound (HIFU) for the treatment of liver and kidney tumours in a Western population. *Br J Cancer* 2005; **93**: 890–5.

7. Wu F, Wang ZB, Cao YD, *et al*. Changes in biologic characteristics of breast cancer treated with high-intensity focused ultrasound. *Ultrasound Med Biol* 2003; **29**: 1487–92.

8. Wu F, Wang ZB, Zhu H, *et al*. Feasibility of US-guided high-intensity focused ultrasound treatment in patients with advanced pancreatic cancer: initial experience. *Radiology* 2005; **236**: 1034–40.

9. Wu F, Wang ZB, Zhu H, *et al*. Extracorporeal high intensity focused ultrasound treatment for patients with breast cancer. *Breast Cancer Res Treat* 2005; **92**: 51–60.

10. Chen S. MRI-guided focused ultrasound treatment of uterine fibroids. *Issues Emerg Health Technol* 2005; (70): 1–4.

11. Tempany CM, Stewart EA, McDannold N, *et al*. MR imaging-guided focused ultrasound surgery of uterine leiomyomas: a feasibility study. *Radiology* 2003; **226**: 897–905.

12. He HY, Lu LL, Zhou YJ, and Nie YQ. Clinical study on curing leiomyoma with high intensity focused ultrasound. *China J Modern Med* 2004; **14**: 37–41.

13. Aubry JF, Tanter M, Pernot M, Thomas JL, Fink M. Experimental demonstration of noninvasive transskull adaptive focusing based on prior computed tomography scans. *J Acoust Soc Am* 2003; **113**: 84–93.

14. McDannold N, Moss M, Killiany R, *et al*. MRI-guided focused ultrasound surgery in the brain: tests in a primate model. *Magn Reson Med* 2003; **49**: 1188–91.

15. Hynynen K, McDannold N, Sheikov NA, Jolesz FA, Vykhodtseva N. Local and reversible blood–brain barrier disruption by noninvasive focused ultrasound at frequencies suitable for trans-skull sonications. *Neuroimage* 2005; **24**: 12–20.

16. Vignon F, Aubry JF, Tanter M, Margoum A, Fink M. Adaptive focusing for transcranial ultrasound imaging using dual arrays. *J Acoust Soc Am* 2006; **120**: 2737–45.

17. Tanter M, Pernot M, Aubry JF, *et al*. Compensating for bone interfaces and respiratory motion in high-intensity focused ultrasound. *Int J Hyperthermia* 2007; **23**: 141–51.

18. Uchida T, Ohkusa H, Yamashita H, *et al*. Five years experience of transrectal high-intensity focused ultrasound using the Sonablate device in the treatment of localized prostate cancer. *Int J Urol* 2006; **13**: 228–33.

19. Kennedy JE. High-intensity focused ultrasound in the treatment of solid tumours. *Nat Rev Cancer* 2005; **5**: 321–7.

20. Gianfelice D, Khiat A, Boulanger Y, Amara M, Belblidia A. Feasibility of magnetic resonance imaging-guided focused ultrasound surgery as an adjunct to tamoxifen therapy in high-risk surgical patients with breast carcinoma. *J Vasc Interv Radiol* 2003; **14**: 1275–82.

21. Wu F, Wang ZB, Chen WZ, *et al*. Preliminary experience using high intensity focused ultrasound for the treatment of patients with advanced stage renal malignancy. *J Urol* 2003; **170**: 2237–40.

22. Wu F, Wang ZB, Chen WZ, *et al.* Extracorporeal focused ultrasound surgery for treatment of human solid carcinomas: early Chinese clinical experience. *Ultrasound Med Biol* 2004; **30**: 245–60.

23. Wu F, Wang ZB, Chen WZ, *et al.* Extracorporeal high intensity focused ultrasound ablation in the treatment of patients with large hepatocellular carcinoma. *Ann Surg Oncol* 2004; **11**: 1061–9.

24. ter Haar G, Coussios C. High intensity focused ultrasound: physical principles and devices. *Int J Hyperthermia* 2007; **23**: 89–104.

25. Rivens I, Shaw A, Civale J, Morris H. Treatment monitoring and thermometry for therapeutic focused ultrasound. *Int J Hyperthermia* 2007; **23**: 121–39.

26. Kennedy JE, ter Haar GR, Wu F, *et al.* Contrast enhanced ultrasound assessment of tissue response to high intensity focused ultrasound. *Ultrasound Med Biol* 2004; **30**: 851–4.

27. Miller NR, Bamber JC, ter Haar GR. Imaging of temperature-induced echo strain: preliminary in vitro study to assess feasibility for guiding focused ultrasound surgery. *Ultrasound Med Biol* 2004; **30**: 345–56.

28. Miller NR, Bograchev KM, Bamber JC. Ultrasonic temperature imaging for guiding focused ultrasound surgery: effect of angle between imaging beam and therapy beam. *Ultrasound Med Biol* 2005; **31**: 401–13.

29. Anand A, Kaczkowski PJ. Monitoring formation of high intensity focused ultrasound (HIFU) induced lesions using backscattered ultrasound. *Acoust Res Lett Online* 2004; **5**: 88–94.

30. Garcea G, Lloyd TD, Aylott C, Maddern G, Berry DP. The emergent role of focal liver ablation techniques in the treatment of primary and secondary liver tumours. *Eur J Cancer* 2003; **39**: 2150–64.

31. Colombo M. Risk groups and preventive strategies. In: Berr F, Bruix J, Hauss J, Wands J, Wittekind C, eds. *Malignant Liver Tumours: Basic Concepts and Clinical Management.* Dordrecht: Kluwer, 2003: 67–74.

32. Lopez PM, Patel P, Uva P, Villanueva A, Llovet JM. Current management of liver cancer. *Eur J Cancer Suppl* 2007; **5** (5): 444–6.

33. Hassoun Z, Gores GJ. Treatment of hepatocellular carcinoma. *Clin Gastroenterol Hepatol* 2003; **1**: 10–18.

34. Crawford JM. Liver and biliary tract. In: Kumar V, Abbas AK, Fausto N, eds. *Robbins and Cotran Pathologic Basis of Disease*, 7th edn. Philadelphia, PA: Saunders, 2004: 924–7.

35. Gazet JC. *Carcinoma of the Liver, Biliary Tract and Pancreas.* London: Edward Arnold, 1983.

36. Colombo M. Natural history of hepatocellular carcinoma. *Cancer Imaging* 2005; **5**: 85–8.

37. Li CX, Xu GL, Jiang ZY, *et al.* Analysis of clinical effect of high-intensity focused ultrasound on liver cancer. *World J Gastroenterol* 2004; **10**: 2201–4.

38. Fry FJ, Johnson LK. Tumor irradiation with intense ultrasound. *Ultrasound Med Biol* 1978; **4**: 337–41.

39. Bataille N, Vallancien G, Chopin D. Antitumoral local effect and metastatic risk of focused extracorporeal pyrotherapy on Dunning R-3327 tumors. *Eur Urol* 1996; **29**: 72–7.

40. Chapelon JY, Prat F, Sibille A, *et al.* Extracorporeal, selective focused destruction of hepatic tumours by high intensity ultrasound in rabbits bearing VX-2 carcinoma. *Minim Invasive Ther* 1992; **1**: 287–93.

41. Oosterhof GON, Cornel EB, Smits GAHJ, Debruyne FMJ, Schalken JA. Influence of high-intensity focused ultrasound on the development of metastases. *Eur Urol* 1997; **32**: 91–5.

42. Yang R, Reilly CR, Rescorla FJ, *et al.* High intensity focused ultrasound in the treatment of experimental liver cancer. *Arch Surg* 1991; **126**: 1002–9.

43. Wu F, Wang ZB, Jin CB, *et al.* Circulating tumor cells in patients with solid malignancy treated by high-intensity focused ultrasound. *Ultrasound Med Biol* 2004; **30**: 511–17.

44. Wu F, Wang ZB, Lu P, *et al.* Activated anti-tumor immunity in cancer patients after high intensity focused ultrasound ablation. *Ultrasound Med Biol* 2004; **30**: 1217–22.

6

Percutaneous ethanol injection of hepatocellular carcinoma

K. T. Tan and C. S. Ho

Introduction

Hepatocellular carcinoma (HCC) is the fifth most common cancer worldwide. The major clinical risk factor is the development of liver cirrhosis, and the most important risk factors for the development of cirrhosis are chronic infection with the hepatitis B and C viruses and chronic heavy alcohol consumption. The current increasing incidence of HCC is due to widespread dissemination of the hepatitis viruses [1]. At present, there are over 200 million people around the world infected with hepatitis C, giving an incidence of around 3.3% of the world's population [2]. Meanwhile, despite the introduction of hepatitis B vaccine, 5–6% of the world's population are chronic carriers of the disease [3]. Most HCCs develop through a progressive pathway from premalignant nodular lesions to cancerous lesions in the cirrhotic liver [4]. The progression takes an average of 2–4 decades from the time of initial infection to cirrhosis. Thereafter, the annual risk of HCC is 2–3% for hepatitis B, 1–7% for hepatitis C, and 1% for alcohol-induced cirrhosis [5–8].

Surgical resection is the current standard modality to achieve long-term survival. It may be offered to patients with single-lesion HCC and well-preserved hepatic function (e.g., Child A cirrhosis). Patients with Child B or C cirrhosis cannot tolerate loss of surrounding non-tumorous hepatic parenchyma during a local resection. Even some patients with Child A cirrhosis (e.g., those with signs of portal hypertension or hyperbilirubinemia) cannot tolerate this loss and are not candidates for local resection. Metastatic disease and gross vascular spread into the main portal vein or inferior vena cava (by the hepatic veins) are also exclusion criteria. Tumor size is not an exclusion criterion, but large tumors mandate large resections, leaving less functioning parenchyma behind. For these reasons, only 5–10% of

Interventional Radiological Treatment of Liver Tumors, ed. Andy Adam and Peter R. Mueller.
Published by Cambridge University Press. © Cambridge University Press 2009.

cirrhotic patients with HCC fit the surgical criteria for resection [9,10]. In patients meeting selection criteria, resection offers 5-year survival rates of 50–70%. However, about 70% of patients have recurrent HCC at 5 years after resection [11]. Adjuvant chemotherapy and chemoembolization have not been conclusively shown to provide any added benefit [12,13]. Various other adjuvant treatment approaches, including internal radiation with iodine-131-labeled lipiodol, adoptive immunotherapy with activated lymphocytes, and interferon have shown promising results but need further validation [14–17].

In 1996 Mazzaferro *et al.* reported that in carefully selected groups of patients with HCC, liver transplantation provided a 5-year survival of greater than 70% with a recurrence rate of less than 15% [18]. Accordingly, the result of this study has become the reference standard or the Milan Criteria for all other treatments of HCC. However, there are two main issues with transplantation. First, only about 30–40% of patients will meet the criteria for transplantation. More significantly, due to the severe shortage of donors, many patients succumb to the illness before receiving the organ, hence accounting for the less than 50% survival when the data are analyzed using the intention-to-treat principle [9]. Because of this, alternative therapies such as local ablation, chemoembolization, and brachytherapy have been used to downstage the disease and also as a "bridging" treatment while waiting for transplantation [19–23]. Although surgical resection or transplantation are treatments of choice, less than half of the patients are suitable for the procedures at initial presentation. Non-surgical therapies such as local ablation, transarterial chemoembolization (TACE), systemic therapy, radiotherapy, or combination therapy can be offered to this group of patients. This chapter will concentrate specifically on the role of percutaneous ethanol ablation (PEI) therapy for HCC.

Percutaneous ethanol injection

PEI was first reported in Japan in 1983 and has become the most widely used ablation therapy until recent years [24]. The principle of ethanol injection is based on its ability to cause coagulative necrosis of cells and thrombosis of the microcirculation. These effects are the result of protein denaturation and rapid dehydration of both parenchymal and endothelial cells [25,26]. It is important to bear in mind that these effects are not specific to the tumor cells or vasculature, and alcohol will cause extensive tissue injury if not used diligently. However, one of the main reasons that PEI is effective in the treatment of HCC is the fact that the majority of patients with HCC have underlying cirrhosis of the liver. The parenchyma of cirrhotic liver is often much firmer or harder in comparison to the tumor, which is soft, with the result that alcohol or any liquid agent injected into the HCC tends to be constrained by the surrounding fibrotic liver parenchyma. In contrast, for the same reason, PEI is not very effective in hepatic metastasis because this group of patients usually has no underlying chronic liver disease and therefore the injected alcohol diffuses into the normal liver parenchyma, leaving parts of the metastasis untreated.

Despite the introduction of many other ablation techniques, PEI remains a safe, effective, and low-cost method of treatment for HCC, especially for small lesions. In this chapter we review the techniques, indications and contraindications, adverse effects and complications, tools for evaluating the therapeutic effect, and short-term and long-term results of PEI treatment. We present our view of its role in the treatment of HCC with regard to other interventional therapies.

Techniques

Pretreatment assessments

A standard staging computed tomography (CT) or magnetic resonance imaging (MRI) is performed to identify the number, location, and size of tumors within the liver. Main or lobar portal vein involvement must be excluded. Ultrasonography (US) is required to assess the feasibility of PEI. The target lesion must be identifiable on US. Conventional chest radiography and bone scintigraphy are utilized to exclude extrahepatic disease. Routine hematological tests are carried out and alpha-fetoprotein (AFP) is measured. Child–Pugh classification for cirrhosis is determined.

Equipment

PEI is best performed under US guidance. This permits real-time imaging not only for accurate needle placement but also for continuous monitoring during alcohol injection. The injected alcohol creates a hyperechoic area that increases with the injected volume. Treated areas become hyperechoic while the untreated segments remain hypoechoic. The needle can then be repositioned in the untreated segments, in the same sitting or in other sessions. Real-time imaging also prevents excessive alcohol leakage into the blood vessels or biliary tree, identifiable as

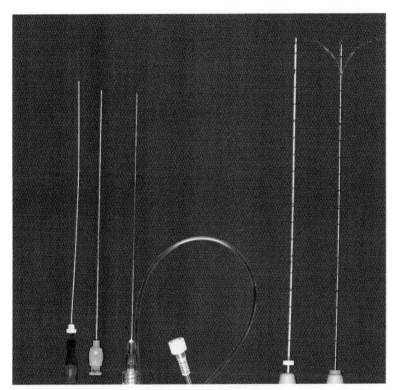

Figure 6.1 Types of needles used for PEI. Left to right: 22G end-hole Chiba needle; 22G side-hole PEIT needle; 20G Bernadino needle; Multi-pronged retractable needle (QuadraFuse needle) with tines completely withdrawn; Multi-pronged retractable needle with tines fully extended.

hyperechoic "bubbles" flowing in the direction of blood or bile. Small leakage into the portal or hepatic vein is usually of no clinical concern. Injection of a large volume of alcohol into the hepatic vein may cause prolonged hypoxemia. Similarly, inadvertent injection of a large volume of alcohol into the biliary tree or portal venous system may lead to biliary necrosis and hepatic abscess or portal venous thrombosis.

There are three types of needles for PEI (Fig. 6.1): (1) 22G end-hole Chiba needle, (2) 22G close-ended multi-side-hole needle, also known as the PEIT needle (Hakko, Tokyo, Japan) or the Bernadino needle (Cook, Bloomington, Indiana, USA), and (3) 18G multi-pronged retractable needle (QuadraFuse; RexMedical, Philadelphia, Pennsylvania). The Chiba needle allows precise injection into small lesions, but in larger lesions multiple needle placements are required. The PEIT or Bernadino needle permits larger volume injection in one needle placement due to the multiple side-holes. The recently introduced QuadraFuse needle has three retractable prongs that can be adjusted for diameters ranging from 0 to 5 cm. It facilitates a wider and more even distribution of alcohol within the hepatoma [27].

Procedure

Generally, PEI can be performed as a day case. Overnight stay is rarely required unless the patient develops severe pain or complications post-procedure. All patients should be fasted for the procedure. Premedication with intravenous analgesia and sedation is routinely administered. Leakage of alcohol into the peritoneum or the liver capsule can give rise to severe pain during the procedure. Prophylactic antibiotics are given only in patients with previous biliary surgery or interventions such as papillotomy or stenting.

The main techniques in PEI are (1) conventional multi-session technique, (2) single-shot method, and (3) injection with the multi-pronged needle [24,27–31]. The choice depends on the size of the lesion, and on the availability of equipment and resources. The conventional multi-session method is the most frequently utilized technique. It involves a small volume (1–10 ml) of alcohol injection per session, repeated once or twice weekly for a total of 6 to 12 sessions depending on the size and number of lesions. Usually up to three injections are performed during each treatment session. The alcohol is injected slowly at a rate of approximately 1 ml in 5–10 seconds. The needle used in this technique is generally the end-hole Chiba needle. In small tumors (< 3 cm) the needle is placed in the center of the lesion in the first session and in the periphery of the tumor in subsequent sessions. It is imperative that the treated segments are carefully documented during each session, to ensure that all areas are treated. The alcohol injection is performed under real-time ultrasound and should be stopped when the target area is completely echogenic, or when there is significant alcohol leakage outside the lesion, or when pain becomes intolerable (Fig. 6.2).

In large lesions (> 3 cm), multi-site injection can be performed in the same sitting to decrease the number of sessions. Also in large lesions, multiple needle placements can be performed before any alcohol injections because hyperechogenicity post-injection often makes subsequent needle placement difficult or even impossible. After injection, the needle must be left in situ for one minute to reduce alcohol refluxing into the peritoneal cavity, which can cause intense pain. Following the

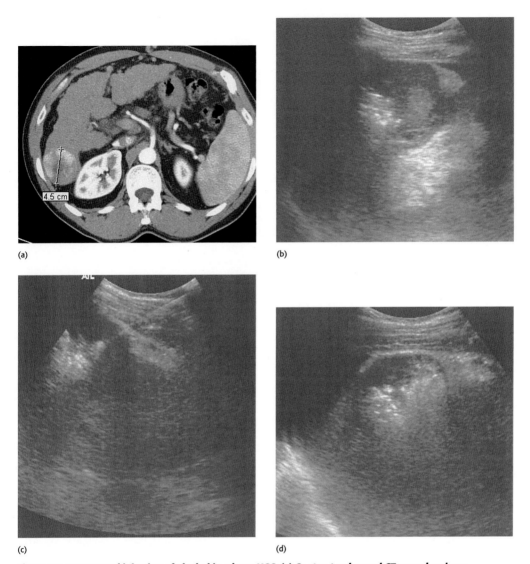

(a)

(b)

(c)

(d)

Figure 6.2 Incremental injection of alcohol in a large HCC. (a) Contrast-enhanced CT scan showing a hypervascular 4.5 cm hepatoma in segment VI. (b) A small amount of alcohol has been injected at the deepest area of the tumor (furthest away from skin entry). This appears as a hyperechoic area. (c) The needle has been withdrawn to the mid-portion of the hepatoma and alcohol injected further increases the area of hyperechogenicity. (d) The hyperechoic area increases to almost completely cover the tumor, except for a portion of hypoechoic area in the near field. Injection was stopped because of pain. This area was injected at a subsequent session 1 week later. (e) Follow-up contrast-enhanced CT a week later: arterial-phase image showing complete ablation of the hepatoma. A total of 45 ml of alcohol was injected in two sessions.

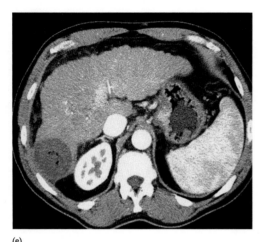

(e)

Figure 6.2 (cont.)

treatment, patients are kept under medical observation for 3–4 hours before being discharged.

Multi-session technique is time-consuming, particularly for a large (> 5 cm) lesion or multiple lesions. The single-session technique was introduced to decrease the number of treatment sessions and also to treat larger lesions (> 5 cm) [28,29]. This technique allows the injection of a large volume of alcohol (40–150 ml vs. 2–10 ml per session in multi-session technique). Due to the systemic toxicity of alcohol and the severe pain that can occur during the procedure, this technique has to be performed under general anesthesia. Before the procedure, the patients are also administered with fructose-1,6-bisphosphate and glutathione-SH by intravenous infusion to minimize systemic toxicity of alcohol. The deep segment of the lesion is injected first via a Chiba or PEIT needle to prevent obscuration of subsequent needle placement. The target zone must be completely echogenic before stopping injection. All patients are hospitalized for 48–72 hours post-treatment and are kept well hydrated to decrease the toxic effect of alcohol.

Using the QuadraFuse needle, a large volume of alcohol can be distributed more evenly in the tumor in one session. Unlike the single-shot technique, this can be performed under conscious sedation. Once the needle is inserted in the lesion, the tines are extended to a desirable diameter for injection. As the alcohol is being injected, the tines are gradually retracted to within the needle. Once retraction is complete, the needle is then rotated 60° and the tines re-extended for another round of injection. In larger lesions, it may be necessary to withdraw the needle to a more proximal location within the tumor for further injection. No more than 60 ml of alcohol is recommended for each session. This needle significantly reduces the number of alcohol injections required for medium and large HCCs [27].

Two methods are available to estimate the total volume of alcohol required for PEI based on the size of the tumor. Generally, the injected volume should be at least equal to the size of the lesion. Assuming a complete spherical lesion, the volume can be calculated by the formula:

$$V(\text{ml}) = 4/3\pi r^3, \text{where } r = \text{radius of the lesion in cm}$$

Some authors recommend that the value 0.5 is added to the radius (r + 0.5 cm) to provide a safety margin of ablation. However, this formula is not completely reliable in clinical practice. The amount of alcohol necessary to ablate a lesion depends not only on the size of the lesion but also on conditions such as tumor consistency (soft tumor retains alcohol better than hard lesion), degree of vascularity (hypervascular lesion washes out the injected alcohol), the presence of internal septae (limit the diffusion of alcohol within the lesion), and absence of tumor capsule, e.g., infiltrative tumor (allows diffusion of alcohol to adjacent non-tumor liver tissue). For these reasons, this formula is useful only as a rough estimate of alcohol needed. Another method for volume estimation of alcohol allows 10 ml of alcohol for each centimeter of diameter of the lesion. For example, 50 ml would be injected in a 5 cm lesion. Ensuring that the lesion is completely hyperechoic post-treatment, however, is a better guide to complete ablation than the volume of alcohol injected.

In our institution, we routinely schedule the patients for three treatment sessions at weekly intervals. Triphasic CT examination is performed before the ablation therapy. The type of needle used depends highly on the size and location of the lesion. Small lesions (< 3 cm) are usually treated with the Chiba end-hole needle or the Bernadino side-hole needle, whilst the QuadraFuse needle is used for lesions > 3 cm. Location of tumor is also highly important. Lesions that are exophytic or located adjacent to other structures such as colon or gallbladder, where precise needle placement is important, are best approached using an end-hole needle (Fig. 6.3). Central lesions, where precise needle placement is not as crucial, can usually be treated safely using a multi-pronged needle.

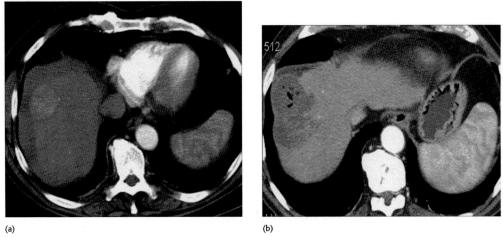

(a)   (b)

Figure 6.3 PEI of an exophytic hepatocellular carcinoma. (a) Pre-injection contrast-enhanced triphasic CT: arterial-phase image showing a 3 cm exophytic hepatoma in segment VIII. (b) Post-injection contrast-enhanced triphasic CT: arterial-phase image showing complete necrosis of the hepatoma.

Indications and contraindications

The indications for PEI can be divided into two main categories: intent-to-treat or as a bridge to transplantation. To be considered eligible, the patients must have disease that is confined to the liver, with no extrahepatic involvement. Lobar or main portal vein tumor thrombus is also a contraindication. Segmental portal vein tumor thrombus is not a contraindication for intent-to-treat but excludes the patient from liver transplant. Encapsulated hepatomas respond well to alcohol injection. However, diffuse infiltrative tumor is not suitable for PEI because the absence of tumor capsule allows the injected alcohol to disperse into the surrounding tissue, leading to incomplete tumor necrosis and also injury to the adjacent liver parenchyma. Lesion size is certainly an important issue. From many studies, a lesion less than 3 cm in diameter has a good outcome, equal to that from surgery or other ablation techniques [32]. Not surprisingly, the larger the lesion the greater the incidence of incomplete ablation and hence poorer outcome. When using the multi-session technique, the treatment of lesions greater than 5 cm becomes cumbersome and time-consuming. Frequently, more than 12 sessions are required for complete ablation. The advent of the single-shot technique and the multi-pronged needle permits the treatment of lesions > 5 cm in one to three sessions.

A cautious clinical assessment of the patient is important when considering PEI. Patients in Child–Pugh C should be excluded, as treatment of the tumor is unlikely to increase survival due to the poor hepatic function [30]. International normalized ratio (INR) < 1.5 and platelet count > 50 000 μL^{-1} are required to decrease bleeding complications. We usually do not offer PEI for patients with more than three lesions, and instead they are offered chemoembolization.

Complications

The complications of PEI for small lesions (< 3 cm) are unusual and are often self-limiting. Mortality of 0.1% and major morbidity of 1.7% was reported by Livraghi *et al.* [33]. Absolute alcohol is highly toxic and induces immediate cellular death when in contact with tissue. The most common complaint post-PEI is pain, either at the treatment site or shoulder pain if the lesion treated is located in the subdiaphragmatic region. Due to the cellular necrosis, low-grade pyrexia is frequently observed in the first few days after the procedure. These symptoms usually resolve within the first week and can be subdued by oral analgesia and antipyrexial medications. With the multi-session technique, elevation of liver enzymes is rarely observed due to the limited cellular death/necrosis. Elevation of the enzymes may be observed if the volume of alcohol injected is substantial, such as in the single-shot technique or using the multi-pronged needle. Portal vein thrombosis is a well-recognized complication of PEI, especially when a large volume is injected (Fig. 6.4). This occurs when there is leakage of alcohol into the portal venous system. In most cases the thrombosis is limited to segmental branches and has minimal clinical significance. Moreover, it tends to resolve spontaneously over the next few months [34]. Hepatic infarction, liver failure, biliary injury, hepatic abscess, intraperitoneal bleed, and tumor seeding have all been described. However, these complications are unusual considering the number of PEIs performed worldwide. Not surprisingly, the incidence of complications is related to the volume of alcohol injected [28]. In this regard, it should be emphasized that serious complications are more likely to occur with large-volume alcohol injections. The mortality is reported to be 0.7% to 2%, versus 0.1% for small lesions, an increase of 7- to 20-fold [33].

Evaluation of therapeutic effectiveness

One of the main issues with PEI is that, unlike surgical resection, there is no possibility of histological assessment of an "excision" margin. Viable tumor cells

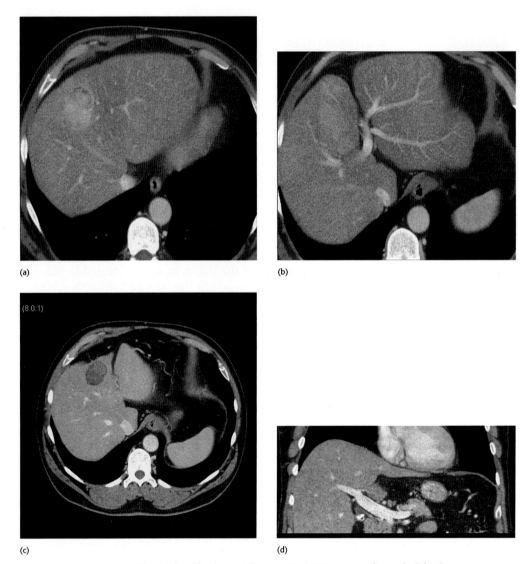

(a)

(b)

(c)

(d)

Figure 6.4 Left portal vein thrombosis complicating PEI. (a) Contrast-enhanced triphasic CT: arterial-phase image showing a 5 cm hepatoma in segment IV. (b) Portal-venous phase showing patent left portal veins. (c) 6-month post-injection contrast-enhanced triphasic CT: arterial phase showing complete ablation of the hepatoma and atrophy of the left lobe. (d) Coronal view of portal-venous phase showing complete occlusion of the left portal vein. The patient subsequently underwent successful liver transplantation, and no residual tumor or vascular invasion was found in the liver explant.

in the margin of ablation are a great concern after PEI. Biochemical markers such as alpha-fetoprotein are of limited use due to the fact that many patients have normal pretreatment levels. Furthermore, the AFP level can return to normal despite incomplete necrosis of the tumor [35]. As a consequence, the assessment of PEI therapeutic efficacy is based mainly on the findings of non-invasive imaging studies. Hence, it is imperative that good imaging studies are obtained before and after treatment. If there is incomplete necrosis, further ablation can be performed.

Until recently, the role of ultrasound in the follow-up of HCC post PEI has been fairly limited, as conventional color Doppler US may miss viable neoplastic tissue [36]. However, the introduction of microbubble intravascular contrast agent allows accurate assessment of viable residual tumor post ablation [37] (Fig. 6.5). Residual neoplastic lesions are characterized by a high and rapid peak of enhancement in the arterial phase followed by a quick washout in the portal-venous phase [38,39].

Dynamic or three-phase CT (non-contrast, arterial, and venous phase) is the most widely accepted imaging technique for the assessment of therapeutic efficacy of PEI. Successful ablation is characteristically hypoattenuating and non-enhancing (Fig. 6.6). Treatment failure is indicated by residual enhancing areas (Fig. 6.7). However, occasionally the liver adjacent to the hypoattenuating area is hyperdense on the arterial phase due to hyperperfusion post-ablation, and differentiation from residual tumor can be difficult. Hyperperfusion is likely secondary to inflammatory response and characteristically appears as a thin enhancing rim around the ablated zone. Occasionally it can also be segmental or wedge-shaped. In contrast, residual tumor tends to be nodular or crescentic in appearance. Another helpful differentiation feature is that hyperperfusion tends to remain enhanced on the venous phase while HCC is unenhanced or shows reduced enhancement due to rapid washout [40]. Occasionally, differentiation between residual tumor and hyperperfusion is not possible, and in this circumstance careful imaging follow-up is required.

Dynamic gadolinium-enhanced MRI can also be utilized for assessment of PEI ablation. Moderate hyperintensity on T2-weighted images associated with corresponding enhancement on contrast-enhanced T1-weighted images offers optimal specificity for detecting residual viable tumor [41]. Viable tumors enhance and appear as nodular or crescentic areas. Similar to CT, inflammatory reaction and hyperperfusion appear as a thin rim or wedge-shaped areas.

The follow-up protocol post PEI includes 3-monthly tumor markers assay and dynamic CT or MRI studies. Further PEI can be performed if recurrences or new lesions are detected, provided that the patient still meets the inclusion criteria.

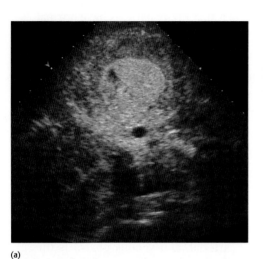

(a)

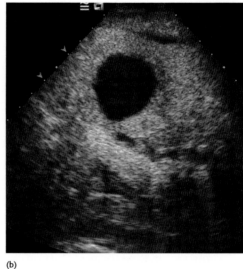

(b)

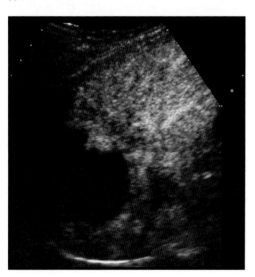

(c)

Figure 6.5 Contrast-enhanced US before and after PEI. (a) Contrast-enhanced ultrasound of HCC in segment VI: arterial-phase image showing hypervascularity of the HCC. (b) Post-ablation contrast ultrasound: portal-venous phase showing complete ablation of the lesion. (c) Contrast-enhanced ultrasound 1 week after alcohol injection of HCC in another patient: portal-venous phase showing residual tumor nodule.

Results

In patients with HCC, the etiology and characteristics of the tumors, as well as the severity of the cirrhosis and the remaining hepatic function, greatly influence the prognosis. Due to the many variables, randomized studies are hard to conduct; hence most data available in the literature are from single-center case series. This

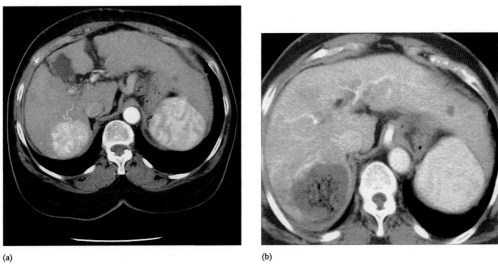

(a)   (b)

Figure 6.6 Complete ablation of a 6 cm HCC in segment VII. (a) Arterial phase of contrast-enhanced CT scan, showing a 6 cm HCC with the feeding hepatic artery. (b) Complete tumor ablation was achieved after injection of 60 ml of alcohol in two sessions: arterial phase of contrast-enhanced CT scan 2 weeks later shows occlusion of the feeding artery, which is no longer visible.

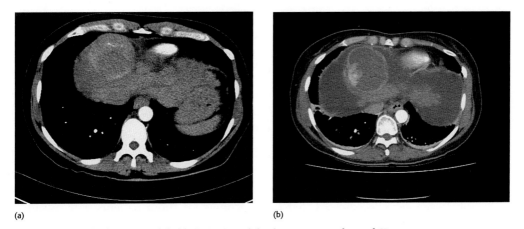

(a)   (b)

Figure 6.7 CT scan of unsuccessful ablation. (a) Pre-injection contrast-enhanced CT scan: arterial-phase image showing a 4.5 cm HCC in segment IVa. (b) Incomplete ablation: arterial phase of contrast-enhanced CT showing residual tumor as an enhancing nodule in the ablated zone.

matter is also compounded by the many treatment modalities available for HCC. The outcome of any ablation therapy is best divided into local recurrence and long-term survival. Local recurrence is an indication of incomplete necrosis post therapy or unablated satellite lesions nearby. Long-term survival is affected by many variables including degree of cirrhosis, residual hepatic function, presence or absence of extrahepatic disease, and also tumor size and number. Not surprisingly, incomplete necrosis is closely correlated with tumor size. PEI can achieve a complete response in 90–100% of HCCs smaller than 3 cm in size, 70% in HCCs of 3–5 cm, and 50% in HCCs larger than 5 cm [42,43]. The reported 1-, 3-, and 5-year survival rates for lesions < 3 cm are 81–97%, 42–82%, and 14–63%, respectively [42,43]. The reported 1-, 3-, and 5-year recurrence rates for < 3 cm lesions are 26–32%, 51–82%, and 60–83%, respectively [42,44,45]. In patients with HCCs larger than 3 cm, the efficacy of PEI decreases significantly [33]. In this series, Livraghi et al. reported that for lesions of 3–5 cm, the survival rate at 1, 3, and 5 years was 94%, 57%, and 37% [33]. In contrast, in patients with nodules > 5 cm, the 1-, 3-, and 4-year survival rates were 85%, 53%, and 30%. Overall, in patients with small HCCs (< 3 cm), PEI and surgical resection seem to give similar long-term survival rates [32].

How does PEI compare to radiofrequency ablation (RFA)? The current RFA devices have the advantages of fewer treatment sessions and also a higher complete ablation rate [46–49]. The complication rates are fairly similar in both methods. RF ablation tends to be more uniform and consistent in comparison to PEI. It does not depend on the diffusion of alcohol and hence is not limited by internal septae within the tumor. In financial terms, the RFA devices cost much more than the needles required for PEI. The cost advantage of PEI, however, can be negated by the increased number of treatment sessions required per patient. Some authors suggest that PEI should be performed in HCC < 1.5 cm in diameter, because complete ablation can usually be achieved in less than two treatment sessions [50]. When the HCC is located in close proximity to major bile ducts or to adjacent viscera (e.g., the heart) PEI is preferred to RF for its safety.

Currently, in those patients with large (> 5 cm) or multifocal HCC not suitable for surgery, multimodality therapy is increasingly popular. Although there is no randomized trial comparing single modality to multimodality treatment, several single-center series showed that the outcomes for those patients with advanced HCC who received multimodality (TACE and PEI or RFA) treatment were considerably better than historical controls [51–54]. Multimodality therapy seems to increase overall survival by 6–12 months. Transarterial chemoembolization (TACE) theoretically treats the small tumors not demonstrable by conventional imaging. In addition, it may also create a fibrous wall around the tumor and hence allow more homogeneous distribution of alcohol during PEI. In our unit, in those patients with advanced non-operable HCC, TACE and PEI/RFA are offered, provided that there is no contraindication.

Summary

Percutaneous ethanol injection is a well-established, effective, cost-efficient, and safe treatment for hepatocellular carcinoma. Its main drawback in comparison to radiofrequency ablation is the inconsistent ablation, particularly in large lesions, and the need for multiple treatment sessions. For this reason it is best suited for small HCCs located in close proximity to a vital organ. In patients with advanced HCC, the combination of PEI and TACE can improve survival considerably in comparison to monotherapy alone. Where RF ablation is unavailable, PEI should be offered for treatment of unresectable HCCs in eligible patients.

REFERENCES

1. Llovet JM, Burroughs A, Bruix J. Hepatocellular carcinoma. *Lancet* 2003; **362**: 1907–17.

2. WHO. Hepatitis C: global update. *Wkly Epidemiol Rec* 1997; **72**: 341–4.

3. Margolis HS. Hepatitis B virus infection. *Bull World Health Organ* 1998; **76**: 152–3.

4. Kojiro M, Roskams T. Early hepatocellular carcinoma and dysplastic nodules. *Semin Liver Dis* 2005; **25**: 133–42.

5. Alberti A, Chemello L, Benvegnu L. Natural history of hepatitis C. *J Hepatol* 1999; **31**: S17–24.

6. Tsukuma H, Hiyama T, Tanaka S, *et al.* Risk factors for hepatocellular carcinoma among patients with chronic liver disease. *N Engl J Med* 1993; **328**: 1797–801.

7. Bialecki ES, Di Bisceglie AM. Clinical presentation and natural course of hepatocellular carcinoma. *Eur J Gastroenterol Hepatol* 2005; **17**: 485–9.

8. Morgan TR, Mandayam S, Jamal MM. Alcohol and hepatocellular carcinoma. *Gastroenterology* 2004; **127**: S87–96.

9. Llovet JM, Fuster J, Bruix J. Intention-to-treat analysis of surgical treatment for early hepatocellular carcinoma: resection versus transplantation. *Hepatology* 1999; **30**: 1434–40.

10. Hayashi PH, Di Bisceglie AM. The progression of hepatitis B- and C-infections to chronic liver disease and hepatocellular carcinoma: presentation, diagnosis, screening, prevention, and treatment of hepatocellular carcinoma. *Infect Dis Clin North Am* 2006; **20**: 1–25.

11. Belghiti J, Panis Y, Farges O, Benhamou JP, Fekete F. Intrahepatic recurrence after resection of hepatocellular carcinoma complicating cirrhosis. *Ann Surg* 1991; **214**: 114–17.

12. Ono T, Nagasue N, Kohno H, *et al.* Adjuvant chemotherapy with epirubicin and carmofur after radical resection of hepatocellular carcinoma: a prospective randomized study. *Semin Oncol* 1997; **24**: S6–18.

13. Yamamoto M, Arii S, Sughara K, *et al.* Adjuvant oral chemotherapy after curative resection of hepatocellular carcinoma. *Br J Surg* 1996; **83**: 336–40.

14. Lau WY, Leung TW, Ho SK, *et al.* Adjuvant intra-arterial iodine-131-labelled lipiodol for resectable hepatocellular carcinoma: a prospective randomised trial. *Lancet* 1999; **353**: 797–801.

15. Takayama T, Sekine T, Makuuchi M, *et al.* Adoptive immunotherapy to lower postsurgical recurrence rates of hepatocellular carcinoma: a randomised trial. *Lancet* 2000; **356**: 802–7.

16. Kubo S, Nishiguchi S, Hirohashi K, *et al.* Effects of long term postoperative interferon-alpha therapy on intrahepatic recurrence after resection of hepatitis C virus-related hepatocellular carcinoma. *Ann Intern Med* 2001; **134**: 963–7.

17. Lin SM, Lin CJ, Hsu CW, *et al.* Prospective randomized controlled study of interferon-alpha in preventing hepatocellular carcinoma recurrence after medical ablation therapy for primary tumors. *Cancer* 2004; **100**: 376–82.

18. Mazzaferro V, Regalia E, Doci R, *et al.* Liver transplantation for the treatment of small hepatocellular carcinomas in patients with cirrhosis. *N Engl J Med* 1996; **334**: 693–9.

19. Martin AP, Goldstein RM, Dempster J, *et al.* Radiofrequency thermal ablation of hepatocellular carcinoma before liver transplantation: a clinical and histological examination. *Clin Transplant* 2006; **20**: 695–705.

20. Otto G, Herber S, Heise M, *et al.* Response to transarterial chemoembolization as a biological selection criterion for liver transplantation in hepatocellular carcinoma. *Liver Transpl* 2006; **12**: 1260–7.

21. Kulik LM, Atassi B, van Holsbeeck L, *et al.* Yttrium-90 microspheres (TheraSphere) treatment of unresectable hepatocellular carcinoma: downstaging to resection, RFA and bridge to transplantation. *J Surg Oncol* 2006; **94**: 572–86.

22. Lu DS, Yu NC, Raman SS, *et al.* Percutaneous radiofrequency ablation of hepatocellular carcinoma as a bridge to liver transplantation. *Hepatology* 2005; **41**: 1130–7.

23. Graziadei IW, Sandmueller H, Waldenberger P, *et al.* Chemoembolization followed by liver transplantation for hepatocellular carcinoma impedes tumor progression while on the waiting list and leads to excellent outcome. *Liver Transpl* 2003; **9**: 557–63.

24. Sugiura N, Takara K, Ohto M, Okuda K, Hirooka N. [Treatment of small hepatocellular carcinoma by percutaneous injection of ethanol into tumor with real-time ultrasound monitoring.] (Japanese) *Acta Hepatol Jpn* 1983; **24**: 920.

25. Burgener FA, Steinmetz SD. Treatment of experimental adenocarcinomas by percutaneous intratumoral injection of absolute ethanol. *Invest Radiol* 1986; **122**: 472–8.

26. Shiina S, Tagawa K, Unuma T, *et al.* Percutaneous ethanol injection therapy for hepatocellular carcinoma: a histopathologic study. *Cancer* 1991; **68**: 1524–30.

27. Ho CS, Kachura JR, Gallinger S, *et al.* Percutaneous ethanol injection of unresectable medium-to-large hepatomas using a multipronged needle: efficacy and safety. *Cardiovasc Intervent Radiol* 2007; **30**: 241–7.

28. Livraghi T, Lazzaroni S, Pellican S, *et al.* Percutaneous ethanol injection of hepatic tumors: single-session therapy with general anesthesia. *AJR Am J Roentgenol* 1993; **161**: 1065–9.

29. Meloni F, Lazzaroni S, Livraghi T. Percutaneous ethanol injection: single session treatment. *Eur J Ultrasound* 2001; **13**: 107–15.

30. Livraghi T, Festi D, Monti F, *et al.* US-guided percutaneous alcohol injection of small hepatic and abdominal tumors. *Radiology* 1986; **161**: 309–12.

31. Redvanly RD, Chezmar JL, Strauss RM *et al.* Malignant hepatic tumors: safety of high-dose percutaneous ethanol ablation therapy. *Radiology* 1993; **188**: 283–5.

32. Huang GT, Lee PH, Tsang YM *et al.* Percutaneous ethanol injection versus surgical resection for the treatment of small hepatocellular carcinoma: a prospective study. *Ann Surg* 2005; **242**: 36–42.

33. Livraghi T, Giorigo A, Marin G, *et al.* Hepatocellular carcinoma and cirrhosis in 746 patients: long-term results of percutaneous ethanol injection. *Radiology* 1995; **197**: 101–8.

34. Bartolozzi C. Portal vein thrombosis after percutaneous ethanol injection for hepatocellular carcinoma: value of color Doppler sonography in distinguishing chemical and tumor thrombi. *AJR Am J Roentgenol* 1995; **164**: 1125–30.

35. Livraghi T, Solbiati L. Percutaneous ethanol injection in liver cancer: method and results. *Semin Intervent Radiol* 1993; **10**: 69–77.

36. Lencioni R, Mascalchi M, Caramella D, Bartolozzi C. Small hepatocellular carcinoma: differentiation from adenomatous hyperplasia with color Doppler US and dynamic Gd-DTPA-enhanced MR imaging. *Abdom Imaging* 1996; **21**: 41–8.

37. Vilana R, Bianchi L, Varela M, *et al.* Is microbubble-enhanced ultrasonography sufficient for assessment of response to percutaneous treatment in patients with early hepatocellular carcinoma? *Eur Radiol* 2006; **16**: 2454–62.

38. Solbiati L, Topolini M, Cova L, *et al.* The role of contrast-enhanced ultrasound in the detection of focal liver lesions. *Eur Radiol* 2001; **11**: 15–26.

39. Pompili M, Riccardi L, Covino M, *et al.* Contrast-enhanced gray-scale harmonic ultrasound in the efficacy assessment of ablation treatments for hepatocellular carcinoma. *Liver Int* 2005; **25**: 954–61.

40. Ebara M, Kita K, Sugiura N, *et al.* Therapeutic effect of percutaneous ethanol injection on small hepatocellular carcinoma: evaluation with CT. *Radiology* 1995; **195**: 371–7.

41. Lim HS, Jeong YY, Kang HK, Kim JK, Park JG. Imaging features of hepatocellular carcinoma after transcatheter arterial chemoembolization and radiofrequency ablation. *AJR Am J Roentgenol* 2006; **187**: 341–9.

42. Hasegawa S, Yamasaki N, Hiwaki T, *et al.* Factors that predict intrahepatic recurrence of hepatocellular carcinoma in 81 patients initially treated by percutaneous ethanol injection. *Cancer* 1999; **86**: 1682–90.

43. Livraghi T. Radiofrequency ablation, PEIT, and TACE for hepatocellular carcinoma. *J Hepatobiliary Pancreat Surg* 2003; **10**: 67–76.

44. Ebara M, Okabe S, Kita K, *et al.* Percutaneous ethanol injection for small hepatocellular carcinoma: therapeutic efficacy based on 20-year observation. *J Hepatol* 2005; **43**: 458–64.

45. Khan KN, Yatsuhashi H, Yamasaki M, *et al.* Prospective analysis of risk factors for early intrahepatic recurrence of hepatocellular carcinoma following ethanol injection. *J Hepatol* 2000; **32**: 269–78.

46. Livraghi T, Goldberg SN, Lazzaroni S, *et al.* Small hepatocellular carcinoma: treatment with radio-frequency ablation versus ethanol injection. *Radiology* 1999; **210**: 655–61.

47. Lencioni RA, Allgaier HP, Cioni D, *et al.* Small hepatocellular carcinoma in cirrhosis: randomized comparison of radio-frequency thermal ablation versus percutaneous ethanol injection. *Radiology* 2003; **228**: 235–40.

48. Ikeda M, Okada S, Ueno H, *et al.* Radiofrequency ablation and percutaneous ethanol injection in patients with small hepatocellular carcinoma: a comparative study. *Jpn J Clin Oncol* 2001; **31**: 322–6.

49. Iwata K, Sohda T, Nishizawa S, *et al.* Postoperative recurrence in hepatocellular carcinoma: comparison between percutaneous ethanol injection and radiofrequency ablation. *Hepatol Res* 2006; **36**: 143–8.

50. Sung YM, Choi D, Lim HK, *et al.* Long-term results of percutaneous ethanol injection for the treatment of hepatocellular carcinoma in Korea. *Korean J Radiol* 2006; **7**: 187–192.

51. Luo BM, Wen YL, Yang HY, *et al.* Percutaneous ethanol injection, radiofrequency and their combination in treatment of hepatocellular carcinoma. *World J Gastroenterol* 2005; **11**: 6277–80.

52. Becker G, Soezgen T, Olschewski M, *et al.* Combined TACE and PEI for palliative treatment of unresectable hepatocellular carcinoma. *World J Gastroenterol* 2005; **11**: 6104–9.

53. Lubienski A, Bitsch RG, Schemmer P, *et al.* [Long-term results of interventional treatment of large unresectable hepatocellular carcinoma (HCC): significant survival benefit from combined transcatheter arterial chemoembolization (TACE) and percutaneous ethanol injection (PEI) compared to TACE monotherapy.] (German) *Rofo* 2004; **176**: 1794–802.

54. Dettmer A, Kirchhoff TD, Gebel M, *et al.* Combination of repeated single-session percutaneous ethanol injection and transarterial chemoembolisation compared to repeated single-session percutaneous ethanol injection in patients with non-resectable hepatocellular carcinoma. *World J Gastroenterol* 2006; **12**: 3707–15.

7

The role of surgery in the treatment of hepatocellular carcinoma and hepatic metastases

Troy Kimsey and Yuman Fong

Introduction

The role of surgery in the treatment of primary hepatocellular carcinoma (HCC) and hepatic metastases has evolved greatly over the last two decades due to the increasing safety of liver surgery and to the emergence of viable alternative treatments, such as tumor ablation and liver transplantation. In this chapter, we will summarize the current data supporting the use of partial hepatectomy in the treatment of primary and secondary malignancies. In particular, we will highlight the evolving and complementary roles of hepatectomy, ablation, and transplantation in the increasingly effective treatment of patients with liver cancers.

Recent reports demonstrating increasing safety of hepatectomy for cancer

When managing HCC and hepatic metastases, the technical advances in liver surgery and the technological advances in ablation modalities have made surgery a more effective part of the treatment regimen in these patients. Recent improvements in perioperative outcomes following liver resection have been well documented. In 2002, Jarnagin et al. reviewed 1803 liver resections including 544 trisegmentectomies, 483 lobectomies, and 526 segmental resections. The median hospital stay in these patients was 8 days, and only 112 (6%) spent time in the intensive care unit. In this cohort the operative mortality was 3.1%, with no deaths in the last 184 consecutive cases [1].

These improvements have also been shown following hepatectomy for HCC. Poon et al. reported outcomes in patients undergoing hepatectomy for HCC in Hong Kong up to 1994 and from 1994 to 2001, and showed a mortality rate of 13.2%

Interventional Radiological Treatment of Liver Tumors, ed. Andy Adam and Peter R. Mueller.
Published by Cambridge University Press. © Cambridge University Press 2009.

in the former group and 2.5% in the latter [2]. Similar improvements in outcomes have been documented at Memorial Sloan-Kettering Cancer Center (MSKCC). Vauthey *et al.* reviewed outcomes in patients undergoing liver resection at MSKCC up to 1992 and found a mortality rate of 14%. Cha *et al.* subsequently reviewed outcomes in patients undergoing liver resection at MSKCC from 1990 to 2001 and found a mortality rate of 2.8% [3,4] (Table 7.1). Similar improvements are seen in studies evaluating outcomes following liver resection for colorectal metastases. Most studies from the 1990s report operative mortality rates of 4–5%, while more recent series have demonstrated mortality rates of 1–3% (Table 7.2).

These improvements in perioperative outcomes following liver resection are attributable to several factors, including improved patient selection, imaging,

Table 7.1 Improvements in operative mortality following hepatectomy for hepatocellular carcinoma

Study	*n*	Dates	Operative mortality
Hong Kong University	136 [2]	Up to 1994	13.2%
	241 [2]	1994 to 2001	2.5%
Memorial Sloan-Kettering Cancer Center	106 [3]	Up to 1992	14%
	36 [4]	1990–2001	2.8%

Table 7.2 Outcomes in patients undergoing liver resection for colorectal metastases

Reference	*n*	Year	Operative mortality	1-year survival	3-year survival	5-year survival
Adson *et al.* [49]	141	1984	–	80%	42%	25%
Fortner *et al.* [53]	75	1984	7%	89%	57%	35%
Butler *et al.* [38]	62	1986	10%	–	50%	34%
Iwatsuki *et al.* [54]	60	1986	–	95%	53%	45%
Nordlinger *et al.* [43]	80	1987	5%	75%	41%	25%
Schlag *et al.* [56]	122	1990	4%	85%	40%	30%
Scheele *et al.* [44]	434	1995	4%	85%	45%	33%
Jamison *et al.* [41]	280	1997	4%	84%	–	27%
Fong *et al.* [37]	1001	1999	2.8%	89%	57%	36%
Minagawa *et al.* [42]	235	2000	<1%	–	51%	38%
Choti *et al.* [39]	226	2002	1%	93%	57%	40%

Table 7.3 Reasons for improvements in perioperative outcomes

- Improved patient selection
- Better understanding of liver anatomy
- Higher-quality anesthetic care
  - Low central venous pressure
- Improved surgical technique
  - Improved instrumentation
  - Improved technical surgical approach

anatomic understanding, anesthetic care, surgical instrumentation, and surgical technique (Table 7.3). Most recently, the favorable safety record for surgical therapy has been further improved by the use of less traumatic and more liver-preserving techniques, including subsegmental resections, combining ablation and resection, and laparoscopic liver resections. The result is that partial hepatectomy, which had been proven for three decades to be a potentially curative therapy for liver malignancies, has become increasingly safe. This modality is also increasingly used in combination with tumor ablation as an effective multitechnique treatment for hepatic malignancies.

The role of surgery in the treatment of hepatocellular carcinoma

HCC is the most common primary hepatic tumor. It is one of the fifth most common cancers and the third leading cause of cancer death worldwide. Its incidence has significant geographic variations, with Asia and Africa having an incidence 5–10 times higher than that in parts of Europe and North America. Known risk factors for HCC include infections with the hepatitis C virus (HCV) and hepatitis B virus (HBV), alcohol intake, and aflatoxin B1 uptake.

Once diagnosed, an appropriate management strategy for HCC includes consideration of resection, transplantation, ablation, or embolization. Since most patients with HCC have underlying liver parenchymal damage, the main factors to consider when determining the appropriate treatment include not only tumor stage but also the functional status of the non-tumor-bearing liver. Many staging systems combine evaluation of extent of tumor and measures of liver function in determining overall prognosis to guide management of HCC. The Okuda classification stratifies patients into three groups based on tumor size, ascites,

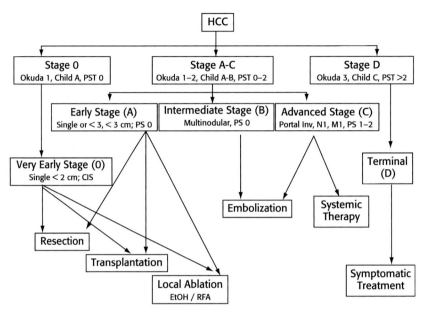

Figure 7.1 Barcelona Clinic Liver Cancer staging for stratification and treatment planning in care of patients with hepatocellular carcinoma (HCC). Child, Child–Pugh score; EtOH, ethanol; Okuda, Okuda Staging Sytem; RFA, radiofrequency ablation. From Llovet JM, Burroughs A, Bruix J. Hepatocellular carcinoma. *Lancet* 2003; 362: 1907–17.

serum bilirubin, and serum albumin [5]. Although this system considers both tumor stage and liver function, it has been proven to be useful in predicting the morbidity of therapy as well as likelihood of tumor recurrence.

Many additional scoring systems have been proposed that have also proven to be useful in identifying patients with poor prognoses [6–13]. The Barcelona Clinic Liver Cancer (BCLC) staging strategy has become a widely used clinical tool for treatment planning. This system stratifies patients into four groups (early, inter-mediate, advanced, and end stage) based on tumor stage, liver function, physical status, and cancer-related symptoms. It has been proven to be effective in linking staging of HCC with treatment planning (Fig. 7.1). Based on the BCLC staging strategy, early-stage patients have solitary lesions < 5 cm or two to three lesions with none > 3 cm. Depending on liver function, these patients may benefit from curative therapy including resection, transplantation, or ablation. Intermediate-stage patients have large or multifocal tumors with preserved liver function and no cancer-related symptoms or vascular invasion. These patients may benefit from transarterial chemoembolization. Advanced-stage patients have cancer-related symptoms, extrahepatic spread, or vascular invasion. There is no known effective treatment for this group. These patients should be offered clinical trials. End-stage patients have major cancer-related symptoms, major impairment of liver function, or severe deterioration of physical condition (performance status > 2). These patients should be offered palliative care. As determined by the BCLC staging strategy, the role of surgery in patients with HCC is usually confined to patients with early-stage disease and is largely determined based on function of the non-tumorous liver.

In general, partial hepatectomy is reserved for patients with good underlying liver function. Consideration for liver transplantation has historically been limited to patients with low-volume disease who are otherwise unresectable based on tumor location or poor underlying liver function. The most widely used criteria for selecting patients for transplantation are the Milan criteria [14]. Published in 1998, these include patients with underlying cirrhosis with one lesion ≤ 5 cm in diameter or three or fewer lesions of which none are > 3 cm in diameter. Patients treated by transplantation have 4-year actuarial survivals of 75%, compared with 3-year survivals of 25% in patients with HCC not undergoing treatment. The survival of patients selected for transplantation by the Milan criteria is not significantly different than for patients treated by transplantation for benign disease.

Efforts to expand these criteria are under way to increase the number of transplant-eligible patients without compromising their outcomes. The University of California San Francisco (UCSF) criteria system is one such effort. These criteria include patients with a single lesion ≤ 6.5 cm or three or fewer lesions with none > 4.5 cm and a total tumor diameter < 8 cm. In a recent experience comparing the proposed UCSF criteria with the Milan criteria in 70 patients, Yao *et al.* demonstrated a 2-year survival of 86% in 14 patients who met the UCSF criteria but exceeded the Milan criteria [15]. In the 46 of 70 patients who met the Milan criteria, the 1-, 2-, and 5-year survival rates were 91%, 81%, and 72%, respectively. In the 60 of 70 patients who met the UCSF criteria, the 1-, 2-, and 5-year survival rates were 90%, 82%, and 75%, respectively (Table 7.4). This expansion of the Milan criteria could increase eligibility for liver transplantation by an additional 20% while preserving an acceptable survival after orthotopic liver transplantation (OLT).

Liver resection is the most common treatment worldwide for HCC in patients with well-compensated cirrhosis. In well-selected patients, hepatectomy can be performed with minimal morbidity and a very low mortality rate. Many studies have shown that patients treated with liver resection have good overall survival rates and are comparable to patients treated by transplantation when evaluated

Table 7.4 The Milan and University of California at San Francisco (UCSF) criteria for liver transplantation in patients with hepatocellular carcinoma

Criteria	Single lesion	Multiple lesions	1-year survival	2-year survival	5-year survival
Milan	≤5.0 cm	≤3	91%	81%	72%
		None >3.0 cm			
UCSF	≤6.5 cm	≤3	90%	82%	75%
		None >4.5 cm			
		Total <8.0 cm			

with an intention-to-treat analysis [16,18–27]. Also, patients with single large lesions who are not eligible for liver transplantation may benefit from resection. Liau *et al.* demonstrated acceptable outcomes following resection of single, large (> 10 cm) lesions [28].

It must be emphasized that, in selecting treatments for patients, the various techniques are complementary. It is not a matter of choosing either resection or ablation or transplantation. It is a usually a matter of choosing the order of these treatment modalities. An estimated 10% of patients with HCC on OLT waiting lists die prior to undergoing transplantation, and the drop-out rate on liver transplant waiting lists is as high as 20% at 6 months [16] and 50% at 1 year [17]. Many liver surgeons, therefore, have suggested that we perform partial hepatectomy on patients with well-compensated cirrhosis, and use transplantation as a subsequent salvage therapy if the patient recurs or suffers liver failure [29]. In other cases, tumor ablation may be chosen for small isolated HCC, and resection or transplantation reserved as subsequent salvage if necessary. Thus, surgery and ablation could serve as a bridge to transplantation and may help select patients with vascular invasion or microscopic extrahepatic disease who are at high risk for recurrence. These patients have poor outcomes following liver transplantation. This form of patient selection may allow the most rational use of cadaveric livers and the most justified use of living-related-donor livers.

The role of surgery in the treatment of hepatic metastases

The role surgery plays in the management of hepatic metastases is dependent on the tumor biology of the primary tumor. Most primary malignancies have the potential to metastasize to the liver, but certain tumors have a greater propensity to do so. For example, tumor cells from gastrointestinal (GI) malignancies spread through the portal circulation to the liver. For this reason, the liver is the second most common site of metastases from GI malignancies – second only to regional lymph nodes. For colorectal liver metastases and for metastatic neuroendocrine tumors, the benefit of hepatectomy has been proven. Use of hepatectomy for metastases from other organs has less firm support and is more controversial.

Surgical treatment of hepatic metastases from colorectal cancer

The natural history of untreated metastatic colorectal cancer has been well studied (Table 7.5). Median survival is 5–10 months and 2-year survival is unusual. Several studies have shown that outcomes in patients with colorectal hepatic metastases are impacted by the extent of liver disease. Patients with untreated solitary metastasis have a 1-year survival of 60% with a mean survival of 25 months [30] and a 3-year survival of 20% [31]. Patients with untreated metastases localized to a single segment have a 1-year survival of 27% [32], while patients with untreated wide-spread liver metastases have a 1-year survival of 5.7% [33]. Hepatic resection represents the only established opportunity for cure or prolonged disease-free survival (DFS). Despite recent advances in systemic therapies, patients rarely survive more than 3 years without resection of their metastatic disease.

Outcomes in patients undergoing hepatic resection for colorectal liver metastases are much improved when compared with patients with unresected colorectal liver metastases (Table 7.2). In 1978, Foster *et al.* published the first multi-institutional data encouraging liver resection for metastatic colon cancer from 99 institutions. The 5-year survival among patients who underwent resection was 22%, versus 0% in patients who did not undergo resection [34]. In 1986, Hughes *et al.* studied 859 patients with potentially curative liver resection and found 5-year actuarial survival rates of 33% [35]. In 1996, Nordlinger published a multicenter study involving 1500

Table 7.5 Natural history of untreated colorectal liver metastases

Reference	Year	n	1-year survival	3-year survival	5-year survival
Bengmark and Hofstrom [33]	1969	173	5.7%	0%	0%
Oxley and Ellis [32]	1969	640	27%	4%	1%
Wood *et al.* [30]	1976	113	15%	3%	1%
Wagner *et al.* [31]	1984	252	49%	7%	2%

patients and showed 2- and 5-year survival rates of 64% and 28%, respectively, in patients following liver resection [36]. In 1999, Fong *et al.* published data from a series of 1001 patients and found a 5-year survival of 36% with a median survival > 40 months in patients following resection of colorectal hepatic metastases [37]. Current 5-year survival rates after margin-negative hepatic resections approach 40%. In studies with adequate follow-up, 10-year survival for patients undergoing hepatic resection for colorectal metastases ranges from 18% to 26% [37–45]. These studies reveal that surgery can cure a subset of these patients.

Once liver metastases are identified, resectability must be determined. The ability of the liver to regenerate has enabled aggressive surgical options. In patients with normal hepatic reserve, 80% of the liver can be safely resected. Historically, the only contraindications to resecting hepatic metastases were the number of metastatic lesions, the presence of extrahepatic disease, and the inability to achieve a complete resection. With improving systemic therapies, the absolute number of metastatic lesions is no longer an unconditional contraindication to resecting liver metastases. Relative contraindications to resection include wide systemic dissemination of disease and/or the presence of serious comorbidities.

Studies have also shown that perioperative outcomes are impacted by the volume of hepatectomies performed at a given center. In the late 1990s, Choti *et al.* [46] and Glasgow *et al.* [47] studied the state registries in Maryland and California and found that hepatectomies performed in high-volume centers were associated with improved perioperative mortality rates, decreased lengths of hospital stay, and decreased cost. In 2005, Fong *et al.* found that long-term survival was better at high-volume centers [48].

Regardless of the institution, patient selection remains a challenge. All patients with metastatic colon cancer are classified by traditional staging systems as stage IV, despite a wide-ranging possibility of outcomes. Being able to determine significant prognostic factors in these patients will allow better patient selection and lead to better long-term outcomes. In an effort to define important prognostic factors following resection of colorectal hepatic metastases, many studies have evaluated clinical and pathologic variables of the primary tumor, clinical variables of the metastases, and pathologic variables of the metastases [19,34–36,38,40,43,44,49–56]. Variables of the primary tumor that impact outcomes are the tumor stage and the presence or absence of regional nodal metastases. Prognostic clinical characteristics of the metastases that impact outcomes are the number and size of the metastatic lesions, whether the metastases are synchronous or metachronous, the amount of time to recurrence (disease-free interval), and the carcinoembryonic antigen (CEA) level. Important

Table 7.6 Clinical risk score and prognostic implications for patients with metastatic colorectal cancer

Score	5-year survival	Median survival (months)
0	60%	74
1	44%	51
2	40%	47
3	20%	33
4	25%	20
5	14%	22

Each risk factor is 1 point: node-positive primary, disease-free interval < 12 months, size of largest lesion > 5 cm, > 1 tumor, carcinoembryonic antigen (CEA) > 200 ng mL^{-1}.

operative and pathologic variables include anatomic versus wedge resections, amount of blood loss and transfusions, extrahepatic disease, margin status, and the presence of satellite lesions. Two large studies have defined these risk factors into clinical risk scores [36,37]. In 1999, Fong *et al.* reviewed 1001 patients and defined risk factors for recurrence following hepatic resection (Table 7.6). In this series, the significant risk factors were extrahepatic disease, margin-positive resections, positive lymph nodes in the primary site, a disease-free interval of < 1 year, metastatic lesions > 5 cm, > 1 liver metastases, and a CEA level of > 200 [37]. These factors were used to determine a clinical risk score for patients with colorectal hepatic metastases. This clinical risk score provides prognostic information and may be helpful in selecting patients for neoadjuvant chemotherapy as well as those who may benefit from PET/CT [57] or diagnostic laparoscopy [58] prior to consideration for resection.

In patients who recur after liver resection, the liver is the most common site of recurrence. It is the sole site of recurrence in 15–40% of patients. In approximately one-third of these patients, repeat hepatectomy can be considered. In patients who undergo repeat resection, the operative mortality is low and 2-year survivals are 23–33%, with 5-year survivals < 10% [59–63] (Table 7.7).

One of the most important developments in the treatment of patients with metastatic colorectal cancer is the advent of thermal ablation in the forms of cryoablation and radiofrequency ablation. This has allowed the use of combined resections and ablations to extend the possibility of safe, complete killing of tumors. This has also provided for a viable alternative to a difficult resection as treatment for recurrences.

Table 7.7 Patterns of recurrence following liver resection and outcomes following repeat hepatic resections

Reference	Year	First resection (n)	Liver-only recurrence (%)	Repeat resection (n)	Operative mortality	Survival 2-y (%)	5-y (%)
Griffith *et al.* [61]	1990	106	–	9	1/9	23	3
Hohenberger *et al.* [62]	1990	105	12	6	0/6	23	1
Bozzetti *et al.* [59]	1992	120	34	10	1/10	23	3
Vaillant *et al.* [63]	1993	189	60	16	1/16	33	9
Fong *et al.* [60]	1994	499	–	25	0/25	30	–

Surgical treatment of hepatic metastases from neuroendocrine tumors

Neuroendocrine tumors are broadly classified as carcinoid or non-carcinoid, and they arise from a number of primary sites including the GI tract, pancreas, and lung. Most neuroendocrine tumors metastatic to the liver are GI or pancreatic in origin. Although GI carcinoids generally have a prolonged disease course, 13% of patients have metastatic disease at presentation, and the overall 5-year survival for all GI carcinoids is only 67% [64]. In these patients, the presence of liver metastases has proven to be the most significant factor adversely affecting outcome, with 5-year survivals of 30–40% in patients with liver metastases and 90–100% in patients without liver metastases [65–67].

Liver resection for metastatic neuroendocrine cancer is attractive for a number of reasons. The natural history of the disease is usually long. The liver disease is often isolated. Symptoms typically correlate with the volume of liver disease. The primary site of disease is usually resectable despite the presence of metastatic disease. The non-cancerous liver is typically normal. In 1977, Foster and Berman suggested that patients undergoing hepatic resection for neuroendocrine metastases may have improvements in survival and symptom relief [68]. Several series have been published since demonstrating low operative mortality, good postoperative symptom control, and 5-year survivals ranging from 40% to 83% [69–80]

Table 7.8 Outcomes in patients undergoing hepatic resections for neuroendocrine tumors

Reference	Year	n	Operative mortality (%)	Symptom relief (%)	5-y survival (%)
McEntee et al. [73]	1990	37	3	88	76
Que et al. [77]	1995	74	2.7	90	73 (4-y)
Chen et al. [70]	1998	15	0	–	73
Chamberlain et al. [69]	2000	34	6	100	76
Nave et al. [75]	2001	31	0	–	47
Yao et al. [79]	2001	16	0	100	70
Jaeck et al. [72]	2001	13	0	100	68
Sarmiento et al. [78]	2003	170	1.2	96	61
Norton et al. [80]	2003	18	0	100	82
Musunuru et al. [74]	2006	10	0	100	83
Osborne et al. [76]	2006	61	1.6	93	40
Hibi et al. [71]	2007	21	0	100	41

(Table 7.8). Recent studies on resection of hepatic neuroendocrine tumor metastases reveal a wide variation (15–65%) in the willingness of surgeons to perform major liver resections for metastatic neuroendocrine cancers [69,72]. Additionally, some surgeons will perform a liver resection only if all disease can be resected, while others are willing to perform this procedure if most of the tumors can be resected.

Although resection for metastatic neuroendocrine tumors is often with curative intent, surgical resection with palliative intent (cytoreduction) may provide patients with palliation of symptoms and prolonged survival if ≥ 90% of the hepatic disease can be resected or ablated [77,78,81–83]. Currently, hepatic resection of metastatic neuroendocrine cancer is recommended if the primary and regional disease can be resected and ≥90% of the hepatic metastases can be resected or ablated. In this setting, 88–100% of patients experience relief of their symptoms [69,71,73,74,80]. In series with long enough follow-up, most patients have recurrence of disease. In 2003, Sarmiento et al. reported on 170 patients followed at the Mayo Clinic for ≥ 10 years. The recurrence rate at 10 years in these patients was 94% [78]; thus, resection is seldom curative. However, the slow pace of growth of these tumors allows resection to have a durable palliative effect.

Factors that predict early recurrence include the size of the largest tumor, the presence of bilobar tumors, and involvement of >75% of the liver [69].

Intrahepatic recurrence is typically multicentric, so segmental ablation or resection is undertaken as the recurrence is recognized until resection is precluded by the extent of disease within the liver. In patients who have undergone resection with relief of symptoms and recur, the median time to the development of new symptoms is 18–24 months [77]. Although cure in patients with metastatic neuroendocrine cancers is infrequent, prolonged palliation is probable.

Regrowth of tumor may require subsequent cytoreduction. Since the liver represents the most likely site of first recurrence, the follow-up of these patients is usually directed at early detection of recurrent liver metastases. Patients with multiple recurrent tumors or those with a short disease-free interval should be offered a combination of medical and ablative treatments. Patients with limited disease and a long disease-free interval should be offered additional cytoreduction with resection or ablation. Ablation is usually accomplished with embolization in patients with multiple tumors, and radiofrequency ablation (RFA) or ethanol (EtOH) injection in patients with a limited number of tumors. These procedures can be very effective in palliating symptomatic patients. In fact, ≥ 90% of patients with symptomatic neuroendocrine hepatic metastases can be effectively palliated with embolization [84].

The high recurrence rates of neuroendocrine cancers after partial hepatectomy have encouraged the ongoing investigation of OLT for the treatment of metastatic neuroendocrine cancer. As with partial hepatectomy, OLT is indicated if the primary and regional disease can be completely resected. Outcomes have been reported in 185 patients with a mean follow-up of 36 months. In these patients, the 1-year survival rates range from 50% to 100% with a mean of 82%, and the 5-year survival rates range from 36% to 89% with a mean of 57% [85–93]. The high rate of recurrence after OLT is, in part, due to poor patient selection. Several studies have attempted to identify factors predictive of outcomes following OLT. In 1998, Lehnert determined that age < 50 years, primary disease in the lung or bowel, and pre-transplant treatment with somatostatin therapy were favorable prognostic factors following liver transplant for the treatment of neuroendocrine hepatic metastases [90]. The heterogeneity of the group studied makes it difficult to know the impact of these factors on individual patients undergoing OLT for neuroendocrine hepatic metastases.

The role of surgery in the asymptomatic patient is less clearly defined. In general, if tumors are large and resectable, they should be resected. If they are small, they can be observed to monitor for progression of disease or development of symptoms.

Surgical treatment of hepatic metastases from non-colorectal and non-neuroendocrine tumors

Surgical resection is established for liver metastases from colorectal and neuroendocrine cancers. Liver resection for patients with metastases from non-colorectal, non-neuroendocrine tumors is not as well defined. Many solid tumors have the ability to metastasize to the liver, including tumors from gastric, pancreatic, renal, sarcoma, breast, skin, and reproductive tract cancers. The benefit of resecting liver metastases in these patients is dependent on the tumor biology of the primary malignancy and is limited to patients with liver-only disease and an interval of time long enough to rule out diffuse liver metastases and extrahepatic metastases.

Patients with metastatic gastric and pancreatic cancers have an extremely poor prognosis. Liver resection rarely plays a useful role in the management of these patients.

Ten percent of patients with renal cell carcinoma develop hepatic metastases, and < 10% of these patients survive beyond 1 year without treatment. Given such poor prognosis, and few effective systemic agents, liver resection has been used to produce cytoreduction. In general, only patients with disease isolated to the liver and a long disease-free interval before discovery of liver metastases are chosen for hepatectomy.

A benefit has been demonstrated in selected patients undergoing liver resections for metastatic sarcoma. In 2001, DeMatteo *et al.* reported on 56 patients with isolated liver metastases from GI stromal tumor (GIST) and leiomyosarcoma who underwent resection. The 5-year overall survival was 30% in completely resected patients and 4% in patients who did not undergo resection. In these patients, a disease-free interval of < 24 months significantly impacted survival [94]. In patients with isolated liver metastases from leiomyosarcoma and a disease-free interval of ≥ 24 months, resection of the liver metastasis is reasonable.

In the subset of sarcomas classified as GIST, resection has particular benefits. Gleevec has been proven to be effective treatment for metastatic GIST. Therefore, liver resections are often offered to patients with extensive liver metastases when all gross disease can be removed following maximal response to this therapy.

Liver resection plays a limited role in metastatic breast cancer. Only 4–5% of patients with breast cancer have liver-only metastases. In 2003, Wyld *et al.* showed that patients with liver metastases receiving only chemotherapy rarely survived 5 years [95]. Even with aggressive chemotherapy, the median survival in these patients is 23–27 months, with a time to progression of 8–10 months [96]. Resection of liver metastases from breast cancer has been shown to prolong survival in a highly selected subset of patients, with 5-year overall survival rates of 22–34% in patients following resection of isolated liver metastases [97,98]. The most reasonable approach to liver-only breast cancer metastases is induction chemotherapy. When the disease proves to be responsive to chemotherapy, and proves over time to remain isolated to the liver and resectable, then hepatectomy is performed.

Liver resection for patients with metastatic melanoma is only potentially beneficial in a highly selected group of patients. As shown by Coit and Allen in 2002, melanoma recurs in approximately one-third of patients who have undergone a potentially curative resection of their primary tumor [99]. Most patients with metastatic melanoma to the liver have unresectable disease due to extrahepatic metastases or disseminated hepatic metastases. In 2001, Rose et al. published the findings from 26 204 patients from 1971 to 1999 [100]. Of these patients, 6.7% (1750) had liver metastases. Thirty-four patients underwent surgical exploration, and 24/34 underwent hepatectomy. Twelve of the 24 had synchronous extrahepatic disease identified at the time of exploration. Eighteen of the 24 patients were rendered disease-free. The 10 patients who underwent exploration without resection had a median survival of 4 months. The overall survival of all patients with liver metastases treated non-operatively was 6 months. The mean survival in patients with melanoma metastatic to the liver who underwent complete resection was 28 months, with a median disease-free survival of 12 months and an actuarial 5-year survival of 29%. These findings confirm that liver resection may be beneficial in a highly selected group of patients with metastatic melanoma.

Effective chemotherapy exists for most reproductive-tract tumors. In 2003, Gholam et al. showed that the development of liver metastases was an adverse prognostic factor in patients with germ cell tumors [101]. In 2001, Rivoire et al. attempted to define guidelines for resection in patients with germ-cell tumors metastatic to the liver. After reviewing 37 patients, these authors found three factors associated with worse outcomes following resection: pure embryonal carcinoma of the primary, liver metastases > 3 cm, and the presence of viable residual disease after chemotherapy [102]. For this reason, only patients without pure embryonal carcinoma and those with germ-cell tumor liver metastases ≤ 3 cm should be considered for resection. Metastatic ovarian and fallopian tube cancers are typically diffuse intra-abdominal processes. The current standard of care for these diseases is cytoreduction to < 1 cm and chemotherapy. If liver resection is safe and provides cytoreduction to < 1cm, it should be considered.

Summary

Over the last two decades, surgical treatments have greatly evolved as therapies for primary and metastatic tumors of the liver. The safety of liver resections has improved to the point that operative mortality is routinely less than 5%, even for patients with cirrhosis of the liver. This has greatly extended the use of hepatectomy both as a palliative and a potentially curative therapy for malignancies. In this chapter we have discussed the most common indications for hepatectomy, specifically as treatment for hepatocellular carcinoma, metastatic colon cancer, and neuroendocrine tumors.

REFERENCES

1. Jarnagin WR, Gonen M, Fong Y, *et al.* Improvement in perioperative outcome after hepatic resection: analysis of 1,803 consecutive cases over the past decade. *Ann Surg* 2002; **236**: 397–407.

2. Poon RT, Fan ST, Lo CM, *et al.* Improving survival results after resection of hepatocellular carcinoma: a prospective study of 377 patients over 10 years. *Ann Surg* 2001; **234**: 63–70.

3. Vauthey JN, Klilmstra D, Franceschi D, *et al.* Factors affecting long-term outcome after hepatic resection for hepatocellular carcinoma. *Am J Surg* 1995; **169**: 28–35.

4. Cha CH, Ruo L, Fong Y, *et al.* Resection of hepatocellular carcinoma in patients otherwise eligible for transplantation. *Ann Surg* 2003; **238**: 315–23.

5. Okuda K, Ohtsuki T, Obata H, *et al.* Natural history of hepatocellular carcinoma and prognosis in relation to treatment: study of 850 patients. *Cancer* 1985; **56**: 918–28.

6. Calvet X, Vergara M, Brullet E, Gisbert JP, Campo R. Prognostic factors of hepatocellular carcinoma in the West: a multivariate analysis in 206 patients. *Hepatology* 1990; **12**: 753–60.

7. Chevret S, Trinchet JC, Mathieu D, *et al.* A new prognostic classification for predicting survival in patients with hepatocellular carcinoma. Groupe d'Etude et de Traitement du Carcinome Hépatocellulaire. *J Hepatol* 1999; **31**: 133–41.

8. Kudo M, Chung H, Osaki Y. Prognostic staging system for hepatocellular carcinoma (CLIP score): its value and limitations, and a proposal for a new staging system, the Japan Integrated Staging Score (JIS score). *J Gastroenterol* 2003; **38**: 207–15.

9. Leung TW, Tang AM, Zee B, *et al.* Factors predicting response and survival in 149 patients with unresectable hepatocellular carcinoma treated by combination cisplatin, interferon-alpha, doxorubicin and 5-fluorouracil chemotherapy. *Cancer* 2002; **94**: 421–7.

10. Omagari K, Honda S, Kadokawa Y, *et al.* Preliminary analysis of a newly proposed prognostic scoring system (SLiDe score) for hepatocellular carcinoma. *J Gastroenterol Hepatol* 2004; **19**: 805–11.

11. Primack A, Vogel CL, Kyalwazi SK, *et al.* A staging system for hepatocellular carcinoma: prognostic factors in Ugandan patients. *Cancer* 1975; **35**: 1357–64.

12. Schöniger-Hekele M, Müller C, Kutilek M, *et al.* Hepatocellular carcinoma in Austria: aetiological and clinical characteristics at presentation. *Eur J Gastroenterol Hepatol* 2000; **12**: 941–8.

13. Stuart KE, Anand AJ, Jenkins RL. Hepatocellular carcinoma in the United States. Prognostic features, treatment outcome, and survival. *Cancer* 1996; **77**: 2217–22.

14. Mazzaferro V, Regalia E, Doci R, *et al.* Liver transplantation for the treatment of small hepatocellular carcinomas in patients with cirrhosis. *N Engl J Med* 1996; **334**: 693–9.

15. Yao FY, Ferrell L, Bass NM, *et al.* Liver transplantation for hepatocellular carcinoma: comparison of the proposed UCSF criteria with the Milan criteria and the Pittsburgh modified TNM criteria. *Liver Transpl* 2002; **8**: 765–74.

16. Llovet JM, Fuster J, Bruix J. Intention-to-treat analysis of surgical treatment for early hepatocellular carcinoma: resection versus transplantation. *Hepatology* 1999; **30**: 434–40.

17. Pereira SP, Williams R. Limits to liver transplantation in the UK. *Gut* 1998; **42**: 883–5.

18. Figueras J, Ibañez L, Ramos E, *et al.* Selection criteria for liver transplantation in early-stage hepatocellular carcinoma with cirrhosis: results of a multicenter study. *Liver Transpl* 2001; **7**: 877–83.

19. Fong Y, Sun RL, Jarnagin W, Blumgart LH. An analysis of 412 cases of hepatocellular carcinoma at a Western center. *Ann Surg* 1999; **229**: 790–800.

20. Fuster J, Garcia-Valdecasas JC, Grande L, *et al.* Hepatocellular carcinoma and cirrhosis: results of surgical treatment in a European series. *Ann Surg* 1996; **223**: 297–302.

21. Hemming AW, Cattral MS, Reed AI, *et al.* Liver transplantation for hepatocellular carcinoma. *Ann Surg* 2001; **233**: 652–9.

22. Iwatsuki S, Dvorchik I, Marsh JW, *et al.* Liver transplantation for hepatocellular carcinoma: a proposal of a prognostic scoring system. *J Am Coll Surg* 2000; **191**: 389–94.

23. Jonas S, Steinmüller T, Settmacher U, *et al.* Liver transplantation for recurrent hepatocellular carcinoma in Europe. *J Hepatobiliary Pancreat Surg* 2001; **8**: 422–6.

24. Kanematsu T, Furui J, Yanaga K, *et al.* A 16-year experience in performing hepatic resection in 303 patients with hepatocellular carcinoma: 1985–2000. *Surgery* 2002; **131**(1 Suppl): S153–8.

25. Tamura S, Kato T, Berho M, *et al.* Impact of histological grade of hepatocellular carcinoma on the outcome of liver transplantation. *Arch Surg* 2001; **136**: 25–31.

26. Wayne JD, Lauwers GY, Ikai I, *et al.* Preoperative predictors of survival after resection of small hepatocellular carcinomas. *Ann Surg* 2002; **235**: 722–31.

27. Yamamoto J, Okada S, Shimada K, *et al.* Treatment strategy for small hepatocellular carcinoma: comparison of long-term results after percutaneous ethanol injection therapy and surgical resection. *Hepatology* 2001; **34**: 707–13.

28. Liau KH, Ruo L, Shia J, *et al.* Outcome of partial hepatectomy for large (> 10 cm) hepatocellular carcinoma. *Cancer* 2005; **104**: 1948–55.

29. Belghiti J, Cortes A, Abdalla EK, *et al.* Resection prior to liver transplantation for hepatocellular carcinoma. *Ann Surg* 2003; **238**: 885–93.

30. Wood CB, Gillis CR, Blumgart LH. A retrospective study of the natural history of patients with liver metastases from colorectal cancer. *Clin Oncol* 1976; **2**: 285–8.

31. Wagner JS, Adson MA, Van Heerden JA, Adson MH, Ilstrup DM. The natural history of hepatic metastases from colorectal cancer: a comparison with resective treatment. *Ann Surg* 1984; **199**: 502–8.

32. Oxley EM, Ellis H. Prognosis of carcinoma of the large bowel in the presence of liver metastases. *Br J Surg* 1969; **56**: 149–52.

33. Bengmark S, Hafstrom L. The natural history of primary and secondary malignant tumors of the liver. I. The prognosis for patients with hepatic metastases from colonic and rectal carcinoma by laparotomy. *Cancer* 1969; **23**: 198–202.

34. Foster JH. Survival after liver resection for secondary tumors. *Am J Surg* 1978; **135**: 389–94.

35. Hughes KS, Simon R, Songhorabodi S, *et al.* Resection of the liver for colorectal carcinoma metastases: a multi-institutional study of patterns of recurrence. *Surgery* 1986; **100**: 278–84.

36. Nordlinger B, Guiguet M, Vaillant JC, *et al.* Surgical resection of colorectal carcinoma metastases to the liver: a prognostic scoring system to improve case selection, based on 1568 patients. Association Française de Chirurgie. *Cancer* 1996; **77**: 1254–62.

37. Fong Y, Fortner J, Sun RL, Brennan MF, Blumgart LH. Clinical score for predicting recurrence after hepatic resection for metastatic colorectal cancer: analysis of 1001 consecutive cases. *Ann Surg* 1999; **230**: 309–21.

38. Butler J, Attiyeh FF, Daly JM. Hepatic resection for metastases of the colon and rectum. *Surg Gynecol Obstet* 1986; **162**: 109–13.

39. Choti MA, Sitzmann JV, Tiburi MF, *et al.* Trends in long-term survival following liver resection for hepatic colorectal metastases. *Ann Surg* 2002; **235**: 759–66.

40. Doci R, Gennari L, Bignami P, *et al.* One hundred patients with hepatic metastases from colorectal cancer treated by resection: analysis of prognostic determinants. *Br J Surg* 1991; **78**: 797–801.

41. Jamison RL, Donohue JH, Nagorney DM, *et al.* Hepatic resection for metastatic colorectal cancer results in cure for some patients. *Arch Surg* 1997; **132**: 505–11.

42. Minagawa M, Makuuchi M, Torzilli G, *et al.* Extension of the frontiers of surgical indications in the treatment of liver metastases from colorectal cancer: long-term results. *Ann Surg* 2000; **231**: 487–99.

43. Nordlinger B, Quilichini MA, Parc R, *et al.* Hepatic resection for colorectal liver metastases: influence on survival of preoperative factors and surgery for recurrences in 80 patients. *Ann Surg* 1987; **205**: 256–63.

44. Scheele J, Stangl R, Altendorf-Hofmann A, Paul M. Resection of colorectal liver metastases. *World J Surg* 1995; **19**: 59–71.

45. Tomlinson JS, Jarnagin WR, DeMatteo RP, *et al.* Actual 10-year survival after resection of colorectal liver metastases defines cure. *J Clin Oncol* 2007; **25**: 4575–80.

46. Choti MA, Bowman HM, Pitt HA, *et al.* Should hepatic resections be performed at high-volume referral centers? *J Gastrointest Surg* 1998; **2**: 11–20.

47. Glasgow RE, Showstack JA, Katz PP, *et al.* The relationship between hospital volume and outcomes of hepatic resection for hepatocellular carcinoma. *Arch Surg* 1999; **134**: 30–5.

48. Fong Y, Gonen M, Rubin D, Radzyner M, Brennan MF. Long-term survival is superior after resection for cancer in high-volume centers. *Ann Surg* 2005; **242**: 540–7.

49. Adson MA, van Heerden JA, Adson MH, Wagner JS, Ilstrup DM. Resection of hepatic metastases from colorectal cancer. *Arch Surg* 1984; **119**: 647–51.

50. Cady B, Stone MD, McDermott WV, *et al.* Technical and biological factors in disease-free survival after hepatic resection for colorectal cancer metastases. *Arch Surg* 1992; **127**: 561–9.

51. Cobourn CS, Makowka L, Langer B, Taylor BR, Falk RE. Examination of patient selection and outcome for hepatic resection for metastatic disease. *Surg Gynecol Obstet* 1987; **165**: 239–46.

52. Fong Y, Cohen AM, Fortner JG, *et al.* Liver resection for colorectal metastases. *J Clin Oncol* 1997; **15**: 938–46.

53. Fortner JG, Silva JS, Cox EB, *et al.* Multivariate analysis of a personal series of 247 patients with liver metastases from colorectal cancer. II. Treatment by intrahepatic chemotherapy. *Ann Surg* 1984; **199**: 317–24.

54. Iwatsuki S, Esquivel CO, Gordon RD, Starzl TE. Liver resection for metastatic colorectal cancer. *Surgery* 1986; **100**: 804–10.

55. Scheele J, Stangl R, Altendorf-Hofmann A, Gall FP. Indicators of prognosis after hepatic resection for colorectal secondaries. *Surgery* 1991; **110**: 13–29.

56. Schlag P, Hohenberger P, Herfarth C. Resection of liver metastases in colorectal cancer – competitive analysis of treatment results in synchronous versus metachronous metastases. *Eur J Surg Oncol* 1990; **16**: 360–5.

57. Schussler-Fiorenza CM, Mahvi DM, Niederhuber J, Rikkers LF, Weber SM. Clinical risk score correlates with yield of PET scan in patients with colorectal hepatic metastases. *J Gastrointest Surg* 2004; **8**: 150–8.

58. Jarnagin WR, Conlon K, Bodniewicz J, *et al.* A clinical scoring system predicts the yield of diagnostic laparoscopy in patients with potentially resectable hepatic colorectal metastases. *Cancer* 2001; **91**: 1121–8.

59. Bozzetti F, Bignami P, Montalto F, Doci R, Gennari L. Repeated hepatic resection for recurrent metastases from colorectal cancer. *Br J Surg* 1992; **79**: 146–8.

60. Fong Y, Blumgart LH, Cohen A, Fortner J, Brennan MF. Repeat hepatic resections for metastatic colorectal cancer. *Ann Surg* 1994; **220**: 657–62.

61. Griffith KD, Sugarbaker PH, Chang AE. Repeat hepatic resections for colorectal metastases. *Surgery* 1990; **107**: 101–4.

62. Hohenberger P, Schlag P, Schwarz V, Herfarth C. Tumor recurrence and options for further treatment after resection of liver metastases in patients with colorectal cancer. *J Surg Oncol* 1990; **44**: 245–51.

63. Vaillant JC, Balladur P, Nordlinger B, *et al.* Repeat liver resection for recurrent colorectal metastases. *Br J Surg* 1993; **80**: 340–4.

64. Kulke MH, Mayer RJ. Carcinoid tumors. *N Engl J Med* 1999; **340**: 858–68.

65. Chu QD, Hill HC, Douglass HO, *et al.* Predictive factors associated with long-term survival in patients with neuroendocrine tumors of the pancreas. *Ann Surg Oncol* 2002; **9**: 855–62.

66. Moertel CG. Karnofsky memorial lecture. An odyssey in the land of small tumors. *J Clin Oncol* 1987; **5**: 1502–22.

67. Proye C. Natural history of liver metastasis of gastroenteropancreatic neuroendocrine tumors: place for chemoembolization. *World J Surg* 2001; **25**: 685–8.

68. Foster JH, Berman MM. Solid liver tumors. *Major Probl Clin Surg* 1977; **22**: 1–342.

69. Chamberlain RS, Canes D, Brown KT, *et al.* Hepatic neuroendocrine metastases: does intervention alter outcomes? *J Am Coll Surg* 2000; **190**: 432–45.

70. Chen H, Hardacre JM, Uzar A, Cameron JL, Choti MA. Isolated liver metastases from neuroendocrine tumors: does resection prolong survival? *J Am Coll Surg* 1998; **187**: 88–93.

71. Hibi T, Sano T, Sakamoto Y, *et al.* Surgery for hepatic neuroendocrine tumors: a single institutional experience in Japan. *Jpn J Clin Oncol* 2007; **37**: 102–7.

72. Jaeck D, Oussoultzoglou E, Bachellier P, *et al.* Hepatic metastases of gastroenteropancreatic neuroendocrine tumors: safe hepatic surgery. *World J Surg* 2001; **25**: 689–92.

73. McEntee GP, Nagorney DM, Krols LK, Moertel CG, Grant CS. Cytoreductive hepatic surgery for neuroendocrine tumors. *Surgery* 1990; **108**: 1091–6.

74. Musunuru S, Chen H, Rajpal S, *et al.* Metastatic neuroendocrine hepatic tumors: resection improves survival. *Arch Surg* 2006; **141**: 1000–5.

75. Nave H, Mössinger E, Feist H, Lang H, Raab H. Surgery as primary treatment in patients with liver metastases from carcinoid tumors: a retrospective, unicentric study over 13 years. *Surgery* 2001; **129**: 170–5.

76. Osborne DA, Zervos EE, Strosberg J, *et al.* Improved outcome with cytoreduction versus embolization for symptomatic hepatic metastases of carcinoid and neuroendocrine tumors. *Ann Surg Oncol* 2006; **13**: 572–81.

77. Que FG, Nagorney DM, Batts KP, Linz LJ, Kvols LK. Hepatic resection for metastatic neuroendocrine carcinomas. *Am J Surg* 1995; **169**: 36–43.

78. Sarmiento JM, Heywood G, Rubin J, *et al.* Surgical treatment of neuroendocrine metastases to the liver: a plea for resection to increase survival. *J Am Coll Surg* 2003; **197**: 29–37.

79. Yao KA, Talamonti MS, Nemcek A, *et al.* Indications and results of liver resection and hepatic chemoembolization for metastatic gastrointestinal neuroendocrine tumors. *Surgery* 2001; **130**: 677–85.

80. Norton JA, Warren RS, Kelly MG, Zuraek MB, Jensen RT. Aggressive surgery for metastatic liver neuroendocrine tumors. *Surgery* 2003; **134**: 1057–65.

81. Knox CD, Feurer ID, Wise PE, *et al.* Survival and functional quality of life after resection for hepatic carcinoid metastasis. *J Gastrointest Surg* 2004; **8**: 653–9.

82. Sarmiento JM, Que FG. Hepatic surgery for metastases from neuroendocrine tumors. *Surg Oncol Clin N Am* 2003; **12**: 231–42.

83. Sutcliffe R, Maguire D, Portmann B, Rela M, Heaton N. Management of neuroendocrine liver metastases. *Am J Surg* 2004; **187**: 39–46.

84. Brown KT, Koh BY, Brody LA, *et al.* Particle embolization of hepatic neuroendocrine metastases for control of pain and hormonal symptoms. *J Vasc Interv Radiol* 1999; **10**: 397–403.

85. Cahlin C, Friman S, Ahlman H, *et al.* Liver transplantation for metastatic neuroendocrine tumor disease. *Transplant Proc* 2003; **35**: 809–10.

86. Coppa J, Palvirenti A, Schiavo M, *et al.* Resection versus transplantation for liver metastases from neuroendocrine tumors. *Transplant Proc* 2001; **33**: 1537–9.

87. Florman S, Toure B, Kim L, *et al.* Liver transplantation for neuroendocrine tumors. *J Gastrointest Surg* 2004; **8**: 208–12.

88. Frilling A, Rogiers X, Malago M, *et al.* Liver transplantation in patients with liver metastases of neuroendocrine tumors. *Transplant Proc* 1998; **30**: 3298–300.

89. Lang H, Schlitt HJ, Schmidt H, *et al.* Total hepatectomy and liver transplantation for metastatic neuroendocrine tumors of the pancreas: a single center experience with ten patients. *Langenbecks Arch Surg* 1999; **384**: 370–7.

90. Lehnert T. Liver transplantation for metastatic neuroendocrine carcinoma: an analysis of 103 patients. *Transplantation* 1998; **66**: 1307–12.

91. Olausson M, Friman S, Cahlin C, *et al.* Indications and results of liver transplantation in patients with neuroendocrine tumors. *World J Surg* 2002; **26**: 998–1004.

92. Pascher A, Steinmüller T, Radke C, *et al.* Primary and secondary hepatic manifestation of neuroendocrine tumors. *Langenbecks Arch Surg* 2000; **385**: 265–70.

93. Ringe B, Lorf T, Döpkens K, Canelo R. Treatment of hepatic metastases from gastroenteropancreatic neuroendocrine tumors: role of liver transplantation. *World J Surg* 2001; **25**: 697–9.

94. DeMatteo RP, Shah A, Fong Y, *et al.* Results of hepatic resection for sarcoma metastatic to liver. *Ann Surg* 2001; **234**: 540–8.

95. Wyld L, Gutteridge E, Pinder SE, *et al.* Prognostic factors for patients with hepatic metastases from breast cancer. *Br J Cancer* 2003; **89**: 284–90.

96. Atalay G, Biganzoli L, Renard F, *et al.* Clinical outcome of breast cancer patients with liver metastases alone in the anthracycline–taxane era: a retrospective analysis of two prospective, randomised metastatic breast cancer trials. *Eur J Cancer* 2003; **39**: 2439–49.

97. Elias D, Maisonnette F, Druet-Cabanac M, *et al.* An attempt to clarify indications for hepatectomy for liver metastases from breast cancer. *Am J Surg* 2003; **185**: 158–64.

98. Singletary SE, Walsh G, Vanthey JN, *et al.* A role for curative surgery in the treatment of selected patients with metastatic breast cancer. *Oncologist* 2003; **8**: 241–51.

99. Allen PJ, Coit DG. The surgical management of metastatic melanoma. *Ann Surg Oncol* 2002; **9**: 762–70.

100. Rose DM, Essner R, Hughes TM, *et al.* Surgical resection for metastatic melanoma to the liver: the John Wayne Cancer Institute and Sydney Melanoma Unit experience. *Arch Surg* 2001; **136**: 950–5.

101. Gholam D, Fizazi K, Terrier-Lacombe MJ, *et al.* Advanced seminoma: treatment results and prognostic factors for survival after first-line, cisplatin-based chemotherapy and for patients with recurrent disease: a single-institution experience in 145 patients. *Cancer* 2003; **98**: 745–52.

102. Rivoire M, Elias D, De Cian F, *et al.* Multimodality treatment of patients with liver metastases from germ cell tumors: the role of surgery. *Cancer* 2001; **92**: 578–87.

8

Image-guided radiofrequency ablation: techniques and results

Riccardo Lencioni, Laura Crocetti, Elena Bozzi, and Dania Cioni

Introduction

Image-guided techniques for local tumor treatment have emerged as a viable therapeutic option for patients with limited hepatic malignant disease when surgery is precluded. Over the past two decades, several methods for chemical ablation or thermal tumor destruction through localized heating or freezing have been developed and clinically tested [1]. This chapter focuses on the use of radiofrequency ablation (RFA) in the treatment of hepatocellular carcinoma (HCC) and colorectal hepatic metastases. Radiofrequency ablation, in fact, is currently established as the primary ablative modality at most institutions [2].

Eligibility criteria

A careful clinical, laboratory, and imaging assessment has to be performed in each individual patient by a multidisciplinary team to evaluate eligibility for percutaneous ablation. Laboratory tests should include measurement of serum tumor markers, such as alpha-fetoprotein for HCC and carcinoembryonic antigen for colorectal metastases, as well as a full evaluation of the patient's coagulation status. A prothrombin time ratio (normal time/patient's time) greater than 50% and a platelet count higher than $50\,000\,\mu L^{-1}$ are required to keep the risk of bleeding at an acceptably low level. The tumor staging protocol must be tailored to the kind of malignancy. In patients with HCC, it should include abdominal ultrasound (US) and computed tomography (CT) or dynamic magnetic resonance (MR) imaging, although in selected cases chest CT and bone scintigraphy may be needed to exclude extrahepatic tumor spread. Whole-body CT and positron emission tomography (PET) or PET/CT may be required to stage patients with hepatic metastases appropriately.

Interventional Radiological Treatment of Liver Tumors, ed. Andy Adam and Peter R. Mueller.
Published by Cambridge University Press. © Cambridge University Press 2009.

Percutaneous treatment is generally indicated for non-surgical patients with early-stage HCC – as defined by the Barcelona Clinic Liver Cancer staging classification [3,4]. Patients are required to have either a single tumor smaller than 5 cm or as many as three nodules smaller than 3 cm each, no evidence of vascular invasion or extrahepatic spread, performance status test of 0, and liver cirrhosis in Child–Pugh class A or B. In the setting of metastatic disease, percutaneous ablation is generally indicated for non-surgical patients with colorectal cancer and a small number of liver metastases with no evidence of extrahepatic disease [5]. Selected patients with limited hepatic and pulmonary colorectal metastatic disease, however, may qualify for percutaneous treatment [6,7]. In patients with hepatic metastases from other primary cancers, promising initial results have been reported in the treatment of breast and endocrine tumors. The number of lesions should not be considered an absolute contraindication to percutaneous ablation if successful treatment of all metastatic deposits can be accomplished. Nevertheless, most centers preferentially treat patients with four or fewer lesions. Tumor size is a very important predictor of the outcome of percutaneous ablation. Imaging studies underestimate the size of metastatic deposits. Therefore, the target tumor should not exceed 3–4 cm in its longest axis to ensure complete ablation with most of the currently available devices.

Pretreatment imaging must carefully define the location of each lesion with respect to surrounding structures. Lesions located on the surface of the liver can be considered for percutaneous ablation, but their treatment requires substantial expertise and may be associated with a higher risk of complications. Thermal ablation of superficial lesions that are adjacent to any part of the gastrointestinal tract must be avoided because of the risk of thermal injury of the gastric or bowel wall [8]. The colon appears to be at greater risk than the stomach or small bowel for thermally mediated perforation. Gastric complications are rare, probably because of the relatively greater thickness of the wall of the stomach and the rarity of surgical adhesions along the gastrohepatic ligament. The mobility of the small bowel may provide the bowel with greater protection compared with the relatively fixed colon. A laparoscopic approach or the use of special techniques – such as intraperitoneal injection of dextrose to displace the bowel – can be considered in such instances. Treatment of lesions adjacent to the gallbladder or to the hepatic hilum carries the risk of thermal injury of the biliary tract. In experienced hands, thermal ablation of tumors located in the vicinity of the gallbladder has been shown to be feasible, although associated in most cases with uncomplicated iatrogenic cholecystitis [9]. Thermal ablation of lesions adjacent to hepatic vessels is possible, because flowing blood usually protects the vascular wall from thermal injury. In these cases, however, the risk of incomplete treatment of the neoplastic tissue close to the vessel may increase because of the heat loss as a result of convection. The potential risk of thermal damage to critical structures should be weighed against the potential benefits in each case.

Technique

The goal of RFA is to induce thermal injury to the tissue through electromagnetic energy deposition. In RFA the patient is part of a closed-loop circuit that includes an RF generator, an electrode needle, and a large dispersive electrode (ground pads). An alternating electric field is created within the tissue of the patient. Because of the relatively high electrical resistance of tissue in comparison with the metal electrodes, there is marked agitation of the ions present in the target tissue that surrounds the electrode, since the tissue ions attempt to follow the changes in the direction of the alternating electric current. The agitation results in frictional heat around the electrode. The discrepancy between the small surface area of the needle electrode and the large area of the ground pads causes the generated heat to be focused and concentrated around the needle electrode [10].

The thermal damage caused by RF heating is dependent on both the tissue temperature achieved and the duration of heating. Heating of tissue at 50–55 °C for 4–6 minutes produces irreversible cellular damage. At temperatures between 60 °C and 100 °C near-immediate coagulation of tissue is induced, with irreversible damage to mitochondrial and cytosolic enzymes of the cells. At more than 100–110 °C, tissue vaporizes and carbonizes. For adequate destruction of tumor tissue, the entire target volume must be subjected to cytotoxic temperatures. Thus, an essential objective of ablative therapy is achievement and maintenance of a 50–100 °C temperature throughout the entire target volume for at least 4–6 minutes. However, the relatively slow thermal conduction from the electrode surface through the tissues increases the duration of application to 10–30 minutes. On the other hand, the tissue temperature should not be increased over these values, to avoid carbonization around the tip of the electrode due to excessive heating.

Another important factor affecting the success of RF thermal ablation is the ability to ablate all viable tumor tissue and an adequate tumor-free margin. It is important to note that surgeons always try to leave a tumor-free zone along the resection margin at least 1 cm wide. To achieve rates of local tumor recurrence with RFA that are comparable to those obtained with hepatic resection, physicians should produce a

360° 1 cm thick tumor-free margin around each tumor [11], in order to ensure that all malignant cells around the periphery of the tumor have been eradicated. Thus, the target diameter of the coagulated area must be ideally 2 cm larger than the diameter of the tumor; this may necessitate multiple overlapping ablations [11].

Effective ablation can be achieved by optimizing heat production and minimizing heat loss within the area to be ablated. The relationship between these factors has been characterized as the bioheat equation. The bioheat equation governing RF-induced heat transfer through tissue has been described by Pennes [12] and subsequently simplified to a first approximation by Goldberg and colleagues [10] as follows:

coagulation necrosis = (energy deposited × local tissue interactions) − heat loss

Heat production is correlated with the intensity and duration of the RF energy deposited. Tissues cannot be heated to greater than 100–110 °C without vaporizing, and this process produces significant gas that both serves as an insulator and retards the ability to effectively establish an RF field. On the other hand, heat conduction or diffusion is usually explained as a factor of heat loss in regard to the electrode tip. Heat is lost mainly through convection by means of blood circulation. These processes, together with the rapid decrease in heating at a distance from the electrode, essentially limit the extent of induced coagulation from a single, un-modified monopolar electrode to no greater than 1.6 cm in diameter.

Most investigators have therefore devoted their attention to strategies that increase the energy deposited into the tissues, and several corporations have manu-factured new RFA devices based on technologic advances that increase heating efficacy. To accomplish this increase, the RF output of all commercially available generators has been increased to 150–250 watts, which may potentially increase the intensity of the RF current deposited at the tissue. Multiple or multitined expand-able electrodes permit the deposition of this energy over a larger volume and ensure more uniform heating that relies less on heat conduction over a large distance. Additional strategies to increase the energy deposited have also been developed. Tyco/Radionics uses an internally cooled electrode design to minimize carboniza-tion and gas formation around the needle tip by eliminating excess heat near the electrode. AngioDynamics/RITA Medical Systems markets a multitined perfused electrode: administration of saline solution – at a very low rate – during the application of RF current increases tissue conductivity and thereby allows greater deposition of RF current and increased tissue heating and coagulation.

The commercially available devices were also strategically developed to monitor the ablation process, so that high-temperature coagulation may occur without exceeding a 110 °C maximum temperature threshold. One device (AngioDynamics/ RITA Medical Systems) relies on direct temperature measurement throughout the tissue to prevent any electrode in a multitined configuration from exceeding 110 °C. Two other commercially available devices (Tyco/Radionics and Boston Scientific/ Radiotherapeutics) rely on an electrical measurement of tissue impedance to determine that tissue boiling is taking place. These impedance rises can be detected by the generator, which can then reduce the current output to a preset level.

Thermal ablation is usually performed under intravenous sedation with standard cardiac, pressure, and oxygen monitoring. To perform a typical ablation, two grounding pads are placed on the patient's thighs. When using the AngioDynamics/RITA Medical Systems device, the needle is advanced to the lesion and the electrodes are deployed either to the initial step of 2 cm or to full deployment (when a multitined perfused electrode is used). The generator is switched on and operated using an automated program. The temperature at the tips of the electrodes is controlled and the peak power is maintained until the average temperature reaches the preselected target (typically 105 °C). After the target temperature is achieved, the curved electrodes can be further advanced – if required. When the electrodes are fully deployed, the program maintains the target temperature by regulating the current. As the tissue begins to desiccate, the amount of power needed to maintain the target temperature decreases. At the end of the procedure a "cool-down cycle" is automatically used. After retracting the hooks, the needle track can be coagulated by using the "track ablation" mode, which maintains the temperature above 70–80 °C.

Despite technologic advances and electrode modifications that have effectively increased RF energy deposition and tissue heating, inadequate coagulation remains a problem in some circumstances, and not only with large lesions. Two likely causes implicated in reduced coagulation include the other two elements of the bioheat equation: (a) heterogeneity of tissue composition, by which differences in tumor tissue density, including fibrosis and calcification, alter electrical and thermal conductance; and (b) blood flow, as a result of which perfusion-mediated tissue cooling (vascular flow) reduces the extent of thermally induced coagulation. These limitations have led investigators to the study of maneuvers or adjuvant therapies in an attempt to improve RFA, either in conjunction with or as an alternative to multiple ablations of a given tumor. In particular, several strategies for reducing blood flow during ablation therapy have been proposed. Total portal inflow occlusion (Pringle maneuver) has been used at open laparotomy and at laparoscopy. Angiographic balloon catheter occlusion of the hepatic artery or embolization of the tumor-feeding artery have also been shown to be useful in hypervascularized tumors [13]. Pharmacologic modulation of blood flow and anti-angiogenesis therapy are also possible but should be considered experimental. Combining thermal ablation with other therapies such as chemotherapy or chemoembolization has to be taken into consideration. The findings of experimental studies suggest that adjuvant chemotherapy may increase the ablation volume beyond that achieved by RFA therapy alone [14]. Further research to determine optimal methods of combining chemotherapeutic regimens with RFA is ongoing.

Imaging

Targeting of the lesion can be performed with ultrasound, CT, or MR imaging (Fig. 8.1). The guidance system is chosen largely on the basis of operator preference and local availability of dedicated equipment such as CT fluoroscopy or open MR systems. Real-time ultrasound/CT (or ultrasound/MRI) fusion imaging substantially improves the ability to guide and monitor liver tumor ablation procedures. Current virtual navigation systems allow determination of the volume of the tumor burden, facilitate planning and simulation of the insertion of the needle, and predict the amount of the induced necrosis [15]. It is important to know how well the tumor is being covered and whether any adjacent normal structures are being affected. While the transient hyperechoic zone seen on ultrasound in and around a tumor during and immediately after RFA can be used as an approximate guide to the extent of tumor destruction, MRI is currently the only imaging modality proven to allow real-time temperature monitoring.

Contrast-enhanced ultrasound performed after the end of the procedure may allow an initial evaluation of treatment effects. However, contrast-enhanced CT and MRI are recognized as the standard modalities used to assess treatment outcome. CT and MR images obtained after treatment show successful ablation as a non-enhancing area with or without a peripheral enhancing rim (Fig. 8.2), which may be observed along the periphery of the ablation zone (see Chapter 3). The rim is relatively concentric, symmetric, and uniform, with smooth inner margins. It is a transient finding that represents a benign physiologic response to thermal injury (initially, reactive hyperemia; subsequently, fibrosis and giant cell reaction) (Fig. 8.3). Benign periablational enhancement needs to be differentiated from irregular peripheral enhancement due to residual tumor, which is seen at the treatment margin. In contrast to benign periablational enhancement, residual unablated tumor often grows in a scattered, nodular, or eccentric pattern [16]. Later follow-up imaging studies should be aimed at detecting recurrence of the

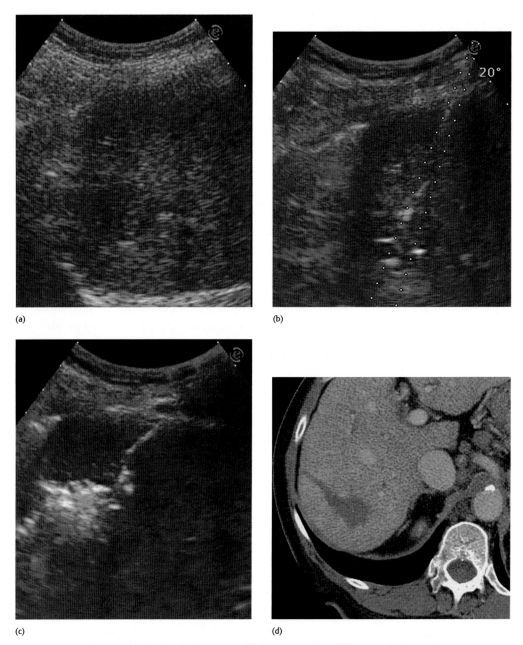

(a)   (b)

(c)   (d)

Fig. 8.1 Ultrasound-guided radiofrequency ablation (RFA) of small hepatocellular carcinoma.
(a) The tumor is localized via intercostal ultrasound scanning. (b) A multitined expandable needle
for RFA is advanced and precisely deployed within the lesion. (c) At the end of the procedure, a large
hyperechoic cloud covering the tumor is seen on ultrasound. (d) Follow-up computed tomography
obtained 1 month after treatment shows an unenhancing ablation zone consistent with complete
response. The ablated needle track is also visible.

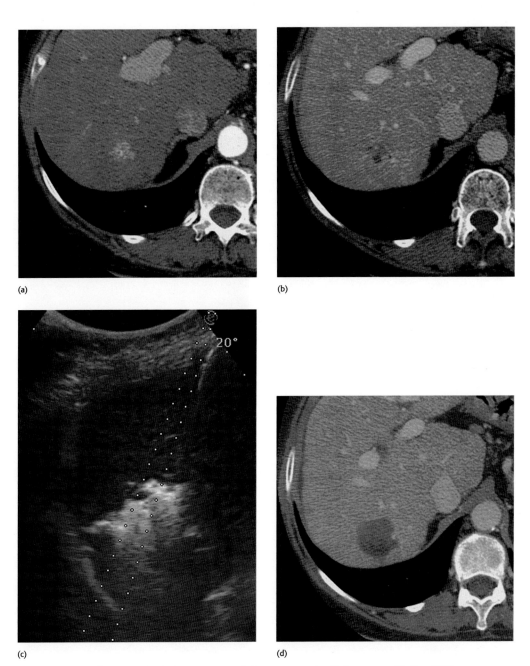

(a)

(b)

(c)

(d)

Fig. 8.2 Computed tomography (CT) assessment of the outcome of radiofrequency ablation (RFA).
Pretreatment scanning obtained in (a) the arterial and (b) the portal-venous phase shows a small
hypervascular hepatocellular carcinoma. (c) The tumor is treated with RFA under ultrasound guidance:
an hyperechoic cloud covering the tumor mass is seen during the procedure. (d) On CT obtained 1 month
after treatment the tumor is replaced by a non-enhancing ablation zone larger than the native lesion. The
findings are consistent with complete response.

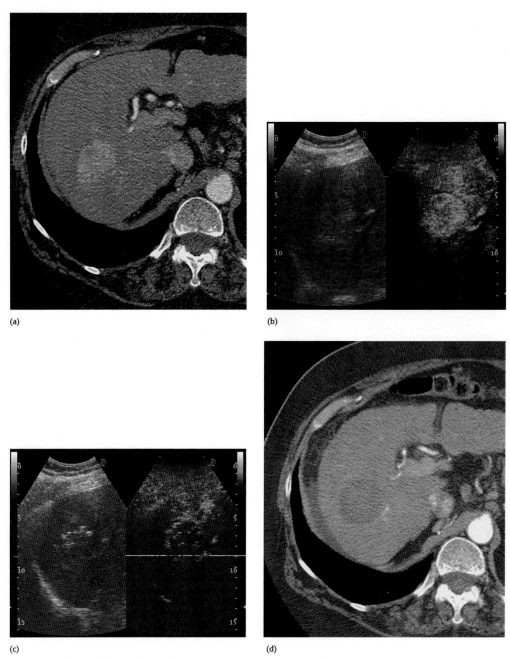

(a)

(b)

(c)

(d)

Fig. 8.3 Contrast ultrasound assessment of the outcome of radiofrequency ablation. (a) Pretreatment computed tomography image obtained in the arterial phase shows nodular hepatocellular carcinoma. (b) Dual ultrasound imaging (left, baseline; right, contrast-enhanced) confirms hypervascular tumor. (c) Dual ultrasound imaging repeated at the end of the procedure shows non-enhancing ablation zone with periablational enhancement. Follow-up computed tomography images obtained in (d) the arterial and (e) the portal-venous phase 1 month after treatment confirm complete response. *See color plate section.*

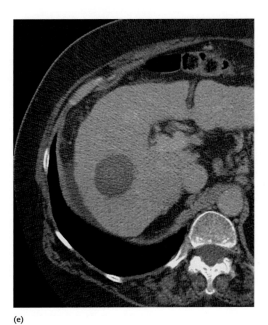

(e)

Figure 8.3 (cont.)

treated lesion (i.e., local tumor progression), the development of new hepatic lesions, or the emergence of extrahepatic disease.

Clinical outcomes

Early clinical research with RFA focused on the effectiveness and the safety of the procedure [17–20]. More recently, the clinical efficacy of RFA has been evaluated in the treatment of HCC and colorectal hepatic metastases.

Treatment of hepatocellular carcinoma

Patients with early-stage HCC should be first considered for surgical treatment, as this may achieve 60–70% 5-year survival in well-selected patients [21,22]. Hepatic resection is indicated in patients with a single tumor and well-preserved liver function, who have neither abnormal bilirubin nor clinically relevant portal hypertension. However, fewer than 5% of cirrhotic patients with HCC fit these criteria [23]. Liver transplantation benefits patients who have decompensated cirrhosis and a single tumor smaller than 5 cm or up to three nodules smaller than 3 cm each, but

Table 8.1 Randomized studies comparing radiofrequency ablation and percutaneous ethanol injection in the treatment of early-stage hepatocellular carcinoma

Reference	Complete response	2-y local progression	Survival rates 2-y	3-y	P
Lencioni *et al.* 2003 [25]					
PEI (*n* = 50)	82%	38%[a]	88%	NA	
RFA (*n* = 52)	95%	4%[a]	96%	NA	NS
Lin *et al.* 2004 [26]					
PEI – low dose (*n* = 52)	88%	45%	61%	50%	
PEI – high dose (*n* = 53)	92%	33%	63%	55%	
RFA (*n* = 52)	96%	18%	82%	74%	< 0.05
Shiina *et al.* 2005 [27]					
PEI (*n* = 114)	100%	11%	82%	63%	
RFA (*n* = 118)	100%	2%	90%	80%	< 0.05

PEI, percutaneous ethanol injection; RFA, radiofrequency ablation; NA, not available; NS, not significant.
[a] 2-year local recurrence-free survival: PEI 62%, RF ablation 96%.

donor shortage greatly limits its applicability. This difficulty may in part be overcome by living donation, but this has inherent limitations and requires a highly skilled surgical team.

RFA is accepted as the best therapeutic choice for non-surgical patients with early-stage HCC. The therapeutic effect of the treatment of HCC has been assessed in studies that evaluated the outcome of treatment at the histological level and in randomized or cohort studies that investigated the long-term survival outcomes of treated patients. Histologic data from explanted liver specimens in patients who underwent RFA showed that large tumor size and the presence of large (≥ 3 mm) abutting vessels significantly diminished the effectiveness of local treatment. Complete tumor necrosis was seen histologically in 83% of tumors < 3 cm and 88% of tumors not adjacent to vessels [24]. Three randomized trials compared RF ablation with percutaneous ethanol injection (PEI) for local ablation of early-stage HCC [25–27] (Table 8.1). The first trial, performed in European centers, failed to show a statistically significant difference in overall survival between patients who received RFA and those treated with PEI [25]. However, survival

Table 8.2 Studies reporting long-term survival outcomes of patients with early-stage hepatocellular carcinoma (HCC) who underwent percutaneous radiofrequency ablation

Reference	Patients (*n*)	Survival rates (%)		
		1-y	3-y	5-y
Lencioni *et al.* 2005 [28]				
Child A, 1 HCC < 5 cm or 3 < 3 cm	144	100	76	51
1 HCC < 5 cm	116	100	89	61
Child B, 1 HCC < 5 cm or 3 < 3 cm	43	89	46	31
Tateishi *et al.* 2005 [29]				
Naive patients[a]	319	95	78	54
Non-naive patients[b]	345	92	62	38
Cabassa *et al.* 2006 [30]	59	94	65	43
Choi *et al.* 2007 [31]				
Child A, 1 HCC < 5 cm or 3 < 3 cm	359	NA	78	64
Child B, 1 HCC < 5 cm or 3 < 3 cm	160	NA	49	38

[a] Patients who received radiofrequency ablation as primary treatment
[b] Patients who received radiofrequency ablation for recurrent tumor after previous treatment including resection, ethanol injection, microwave ablation, and transarterial embolization

advantages were identified in a subgroup analysis of a trial carried out in Taiwan [26] and in a Japanese study, although in the latter the survival benefit was not confirmed in the subgroup analysis of patients with solitary tumors [27]. All three investigations showed that RFA had a higher local anti-cancer effect than PEI, leading to better local control of the disease. RFA is the preferred method of percutaneous treatment in patients with early-stage HCC, as it achieves more consistent local tumor control.

The long-term survival of RFA-treated patients is shown in Table 8.2. In the first published report, 206 patients with early-stage HCC who were not candidates for resection or transplantation were enrolled in a prospective, intention-to-treat clinical trial [28]. RFA was considered as the first-line non-surgical treatment and was actually performed in 187 (91%) of 206 patients. Nineteen (9%) of 206 patients had to be excluded from RF treatment because of the unfavorable location of the tumor. In patients who underwent RFA, survival depended on the severity of the underlying cirrhosis and the number of tumors. Patients in Child–Pugh class

A with solitary HCC had a 5-year survival rate of 61%. Three other studies confirmed that survival of patients with well-compensated cirrhosis bearing early-stage HCC ranges between 43% and 64% [29–31]. In a randomized trial of RFA versus surgical resection in patients with solitary HCC smaller than 5 cm in diameter, there were no differences in overall survival rates and cumulative recurrence-free survival rates [32].

Several questions concerning image-guided RFA in HCC treatment remain unanswered. Some authors have reported that RFA may be a safe and effective bridge to liver transplantation [24]. However, randomized studies would be needed to determine the advantages and disadvantages of RFA with respect to chemoembolization for HCC patients awaiting transplantation. Recent studies have reported encouraging initial results in the treatment of intermediate-size HCC lesions with a combination of RFA and balloon catheter occlusion of the hepatic artery or prior chemoembolization [33–35]. It has been shown that – under the same conditions – the area coagulated by RFA after occlusion of arterial tumor blood supply is significantly larger than that achieved with standard RFA [36]. However, the evidence of clinical benefit associated with this approach is weak, as no randomized trial has so far been conducted.

Treatment of colorectal hepatic metastases

Hepatic metastases are frequently seen in patients with colorectal cancer (CRC). It has been estimated that over one-half of patients who die of colorectal cancer have liver metastases at autopsy, and that metastatic liver disease is the cause of death in the majority of these patients. Surgery is established as the standard of care for CRC metastases isolated to the liver. Recent reports have shown 5-year survival rates following resection of hepatic colorectal metastases exceeding 50% [5]. Unfortunately, only a minority of the patients are suitable candidates for resection, because of associated extrahepatic disease, the extent and location of the lesions in the liver, or concurrent medical conditions.

Many studies have investigated the use of RFA in the treatment of limited hepatic metastatic disease in patients excluded from surgery. Two early studies reported rates of complete response that did not exceed 60–70% [17,18]. Following advances in RFA technique, the reported rates of successful local tumor control following RF treatment substantially increased. In two series, RFA allowed eradication of 91% of 100 metastases and 97% of 74 metastases, respectively [36,37]. The results of RFA in non-surgical patients with hepatic colorectal metastases are shown in

Table 8.3. Studies reporting long-term survival outcomes of patients with colorectal hepatic metastases who underwent radiofrequency ablation

Reference	Patients (*n*)	Survival rates (%)		
		1-y	3-y	5-y
Solbiati *et al.* 2001 [38]	117	93	46	NA
Lencioni *et al.* 2004 [39]	423	86	47	24
Gillams *et al.* 2004 [40]	73	99	58	30
Jackobs *et al.* 2006 [41]	68	NA	68	NA
Sorensen *et al.* 2007 [42]	102	96	64	44
Siperstein *et al.* 2007 [43]	234	NA	20	18

NA, not available

Table 8.3 [38–43]. In three series involving patients with five or fewer lesions, each 5 cm or less in diameter, the 5-year survival rate ranged from 24% to 44% [39,40,42]. These figures are substantially higher than those obtained with any chemotherapy regimens, and provide indirect evidence that RFA therapy improves survival in patients with limited hepatic metastatic disease.

Recent studies analyzed the role of RFA with respect to surgical resection. In one study, 418 patients with colorectal metastases isolated to the liver were treated with hepatic resection, RFA plus resection, RFA only, or chemotherapy only. Overall survival for patients treated with RFA plus resection or RFA only was greater than for those treated with chemotherapy alone. However, overall survival was highest after resection: 4-year survival rates after resection, RFA plus resection, and RFA only were 65%, 36%, and 22%, respectively [44]. In another study, there was no difference in the outcome of patients with solitary colorectal liver metastasis treated with surgery or with RFA: the survival rate at 3 years was 55% for patients treated with surgery and 52% for those who underwent RFA [45]. Other authors used RFA instead of repeated resection for the treatment of liver tumor recurrence after partial hepatectomy [46]. The potential role of performing RFA during the interval between diagnosis and resection as part of a "test-of-time" management approach was investigated [47]. Eighty-eight consecutive patients with colorectal liver metastases who were potential candidates for surgery were treated with RFA. Among the 53 patients in whom complete tumor ablation was achieved after RF treatment, 98% were spared surgical resection because they remained free of disease or because they developed additional metastases leading to unresectability. No patient in whom RF treatment failed to achieve complete tumor ablation became unresectable due to growth of the treated metastases.

Complications

Recently, three separate multicenter surveys have reported acceptable morbidity and mortality rates for RFA. The mortality rate ranged from 0.1% to 0.5%, the major complication rate ranged from 2.2% to 3.1%, and the minor complication rate ranged from 5% to 8.9% [48]. The most common causes of death were sepsis, hepatic failure, colon perforation, and portal vein thrombosis, while the most common complications were intraperitoneal bleeding, hepatic abscess, bile duct injury, hepatic decompensation, and grounding-pad burns [49–51]. Minor complications and side effects were usually transient and self-limiting. An uncommon late complication of RFA can be tumor seeding along the needle track. In patients with HCC, tumor seeding occurred in 8 (0.5%) of 1610 cases in a multicenter survey [49] and in 1 (0.5%) of 187 cases in a single-institution series [28]. Lesions with subcapsular location and an invasive tumoral pattern seem to predispose to this complication [52]. While these data indicate that RFA is a relatively safe procedure, a careful assessment of the risks and benefits associated with the treatment has to be made in each individual patient by a multidisciplinary team.

Summary

The development of image-guided percutaneous techniques for local tumor ablation has been one of the major advances in the treatment of liver malignancies. Over the past two decades, several methods for chemical or thermal tumor destruction have been clinically tested. Among these methods, radiofrequency ablation (RFA) is currently established as the primary ablative modality at most institutions. RFA is accepted as the best therapeutic choice for patients with early-stage hepatocellular carcinoma (HCC) when liver transplantation or surgical resection are not suitable options. In addition, RFA is emerging as a viable alternative to surgery for inoperable patients with limited hepatic metastatic disease, especially from colorectal cancer. Several series have shown that RFA can result in complete tumor eradication in properly selected candidates, and have provided indirect evidence that the treatment improves survival. In this chapter, we review techniques, indications, and clinical results of percutaneous RFA in the treatment of HCC and colorectal hepatic metastases.

REFERENCES

1. Lencioni R, Crocetti L. A critical appraisal of the literature on local ablative therapies for hepatocellular carcinoma. *Clin Liver Dis* 2005; **9**: 301–14.

2. Lencioni R, Crocetti L. Radiofrequency ablation of liver cancer. *Tech Vasc Interv Radiol* 2007; **10**: 38–46.

3. Llovet JM, Burroughs A, Bruix J. Hepatocellular carcinoma. *Lancet* 2003; **362**: 1907–17.

4. Lencioni R, Cioni D, Crocetti L, Bartolozzi C. Percutaneous ablation of hepatocellular carcinoma: state-of-the-art. *Liver Transpl* 2004; **10**: S91–7.

5. Lencioni R, Cioni D. Percutaneous methods for ablation of hepatic neoplasms. In: Blumgart LH, ed. *Surgery of the Liver, Biliary Tract, and Pancreas*, 4th edn. Philadelphia, PA: Saunders, 2007: 1269–77.

6. Lencioni R, Crocetti L, Cioni R, *et al.* Radiofrequency ablation of lung malignancies: where do we stand? *Cardiovasc Intervent Radiol* 2004; **27**: 581–90.

7. Berber E, Pelley R, Siperstein AE. Predictors of survival after radiofrequency thermal ablation of colorectal cancer metastases to the liver: a prospective study. *J Clin Oncol* 2005; **23**: 1358–64.

8. Rhim H, Dodd GD 3rd, Chintapalli KN, *et al.* Radiofrequency thermal ablation of abdominal tumors: lessons learned from complications. *Radiographics* 2004; **24**: 41–5.

9. Chopra S, Dodd GD 3rd, Chanin MP, Chintapalli KN. Radiofrequency ablation of hepatic tumors adjacent to the gallbladder: feasibility and safety. *AJR Am J Roentgenol* 2003; **180**: 697–701.

10. Goldberg SN, Gazelle GS, Mueller PR. Thermal ablation therapy for focal malignancies: a unified approach to underlying principles, techniques, and diagnostic imaging guidance. *AJR Am J Roentgenol* 2000; **174**: 323–31.

11. Dodd GD 3rd, Frank MS, Aribandi M, *et al.* Radiofrequency thermal ablation: computer analysis of the size of the thermal injury created by overlapping ablations. *AJR Am J Roentgenol* 2001; **177**: 777–82.

12. Pennes HH. Analysis of tissue and arterial blood temperatures in the resting human forearm. *J Appl Physiol* 1948; **1**: 93–122.

13. Rossi S, Garbagnati F, Lencioni R, *et al.* Percutaneous radio-frequency thermal ablation of nonresectable hepatocellular carcinoma after occlusion of tumor blood supply. *Radiology* 2000; **217**: 119–26.

14. Goldberg SN, Saldinger PF, Gazelle GS, *et al.* Percutaneous tumor ablation: increased necrosis with combined radio-frequency ablation and intratumoral doxorubicin injection in a rat breast tumor model. *Radiology* 2001; **220**: 420–7.

15. Crocetti L, Lencioni R, De Beni S, *et al.* Targeting liver lesions for radiofrequency ablation: an experimental feasibility study using a CT-US fusion imaging system. *Invest Radiol* 2008; **43**: 33–9.

16. Goldberg SN, Charboneau JW, Dodd GD 3rd, *et al.* International Working Group on Image-Guided Tumor Ablation. Image-guided tumor ablation: proposal for standardization of terms and reporting criteria. *Radiology* 2003; **228**: 335–45.

17. Solbiati L, Goldberg SN, Ierace T, et al. Hepatic metastases: percutaneous radio-frequency ablation with cooled-tip electrodes. *Radiology* 1997; **205**: 367–73.

18. Lencioni R, Goletti O, Armillotta N, *et al.* Radio-frequency thermal ablation of liver metastases with a cooled-tip electrode needle: results of a pilot clinical trial. *Eur Radiol* 1998; **8**: 1205–11.

19. Curley SA, Izzo F, Delrio P, *et al.* Radiofrequency ablation of unresectable primary and metastatic malignancies: results in 123 patients. *Ann Surg* 1999; **230**: 1–8.

20. Wood TF, Rose DM, Chung M, *et al.* Radiofrequency ablation of 231 unresectable hepatic tumors: indications, limitations, and complications. *Ann Surg Oncol* 2000; **7**: 593–600.

21. Bruix J, Sherman M, Llovet JM, *et al.* EASL Panel of Experts on HCC. Clinical management of hepatocellular carcinoma. Conclusions of the Barcelona-2000 EASL conference. European Association for the Study of the Liver. *J Hepatol* 2001; **35**: 421–30.

22. Bruix J, Sherman M. Management of hepatocellular carcinoma. *Hepatology* 2005; **42**: 1208–36.

23. Llovet JM, Fuster J, Bruix J. Intention-to-treat analysis of surgical treatment for early hepatocellular carcinoma: resection versus transplantation. *Hepatology* 1999; **30**: 1434–40.

24. Lu DS, Yu NC, Raman SS, *et al.* Radiofrequency ablation of hepatocellular carcinoma: treatment success as defined by histologic examination of the explanted liver. *Radiology* 2005; **234**: 954–60.

25. Lencioni R, Allgaier HP, Cioni D, *et al.* Small hepatocellular carcinoma in cirrhosis: randomized comparison of radiofrequency thermal ablation versus percutaneous ethanol injection. *Radiology* 2003; **228**: 235–40.

26. Lin SM, Lin CJ, Lin CC, *et al.* Radiofrequency ablation improves prognosis compared with ethanol injection for hepatocellular carcinoma < or = 4 cm. *Gastroenterology* 2004; **127**: 1714–23.

27. Shiina S, Teratani T, Obi S, *et al.* A randomized controlled trial of radiofrequency ablation versus ethanol injection for small hepatocellular carcinoma. *Gastroenterology* 2005; **129**: 122–30.

28. Lencioni R, Cioni D, Crocetti L, *et al.* Early-stage hepatocellular carcinoma in cirrhosis: long-term results of percutaneous image-guided radiofrequency ablation. *Radiology* 2005; **234**: 961–7.

29. Tateishi R, Shiina S, Teratani T, *et al.* Percutaneous radiofrequency ablation for hepatocellular carcinoma. *Cancer* 2005; **103**: 1201–9.

30. Cabassa P, Donato F, Simeone F, *et al.* Radiofrequency ablation of hepatocellular carcinoma: long-term experience with expandable needle electrodes. *AJR Am J Roentgenol* 2006; **185**: S316–21.

31. Choi D, Lim HK, Rhim H, *et al.* Percutaneous radiofrequency ablation for early-stage hepatocellular carcinoma as a first-line treatment: long-term results and prognostic factors in a large single-institution series. *Eur Radiol* 2007; **17**: 684–92.

32. Chen MS, Li JQ, Zheng Y, *et al.* A prospective randomized trial comparing percutaneous local ablative therapy and partial hepatectomy for small hepatocellular carcinoma. *Ann Surg* 2006; **243**: 321–8.

33. Veltri A, Moretto P, Doriguzzi A, *et al.* Radiofrequency thermal ablation (RFA) after transarterial chemoembolization (TACE) as a combined therapy for unresectable non-early hepatocellular carcinoma (HCC). *Eur Radiol* 2006; **16**: 661–9.

34. Helmberger T, Dogan S, Straub G, *et al.* Liver resection or combined chemoembolization and radiofrequency ablation improve survival in patients with hepatocellular carcinoma. *Digestion* 2007; **75**: 104–12.

35. Yamasaki T, Kurokawa F, Shirahashi H, *et al.* Percutaneous radiofrequency ablation therapy for patients with hepatocellular carcinoma during occlusion of hepatic blood flow: comparison with standard percutaneous radiofrequency ablation therapy. *Cancer* 2002; **95**: 2353–60.

36. De Baere T, Elias D, Dromain C, *et al.* Radiofrequency ablation of 100 hepatic metastases with a mean follow-up of more than 1 year. *AJR Am J Roentgenol* 2000; **175**: 1619–25.

37. Helmberger T, Holzknecht N, Schopf U, *et al.* [Radiofrequency ablation of liver metastases: technique and initial results.] *Radiologe* 2001; **41**: 69–76.

38. Solbiati L, Livraghi T, Goldberg SN, *et al.* Percutaneous radio-frequency ablation of hepatic metastases from colorectal cancer: long-term results in 117 patients. *Radiology* 2001; **221**: 159–66.

39. Lencioni R, Crocetti L, Cioni D, *et al.* Percutaneous radiofrequency ablation of hepatic colorectal metastases: technique, indications, results, and new promises. *Invest Radiol* 2004; **39**: 689–97.

40. Gillams AR, Lees WR. Radio-frequency ablation of colorectal liver metastases in 167 patients. *Eur Radiol* 2004; **14**: 2261–7.

41. Jackobs TF, Hoffmann RT, Trumm C, *et al.* Radiofrequency ablation of colorectal liver metastases: mid-term results in 68 patients. *Anticancer Res* 2006; **26**: 671–80.

42. Sorensen SM, Mortensen FV, Nielsen DT. Radiofrequency ablation of colorectal liver metastases: long-term survival. *Acta Radiol* 2007; **48**: 253–8.

43. Siperstein AE, Berber E, Ballem N, Parikh RT. Survival after radiofrequency ablation of colorectal liver metastases: 10-year experience. *Ann Surg* 2007; **246**: 559–67.

44. Abdalla EK, Vauthey JN, Ellis LM, *et al.* Recurrence and outcomes following hepatic resection, radiofrequency ablation, and combined resection/ablation for colorectal liver metastases. *Ann Surg* 2004; **239**: 818–25.

45. Oshowo A, Gillams A, Harrison E, *et al.* Comparison of resection and radiofrequency ablation for treatment of solitary colorectal liver metastases. *Br J Surg* 2003; **90**: 1240–3.

46. Elias D, De Baere T, Smayra T, *et al.* Percutaneous radiofrequency thermoablation as an alternative to surgery for treatment of liver tumour recurrence after hepatectomy. *Br J Surg* 2002; **89**: 752–6.

47. Livraghi T, Solbiati L, Meloni F, *et al.* Percutaneous radiofrequency ablation of liver metastases in potential candidates for resection: the "test-of-time approach". *Cancer* 2003; **97**: 3027–35.

48. Rhim H. Complications of radiofrequency ablation in hepatocellular carcinoma. *Abdom Imaging* 2005; **30**: 409–18.

49. Livraghi T, Solbiati L, Meloni MF, *et al.* Treatment of focal liver tumors with percutaneous radio-frequency ablation: complications encountered in a multicenter study. *Radiology* 2003; **226**: 441–51.

50. De Baere T, Risse O, Kuoch V, *et al.* Adverse events during radiofrequency treatment of 582 hepatic tumors. *AJR Am J Roentgenol* 2003; **181**: 695–700.

51. Bleicher RJ, Allegra DP, Nora DT, *et al.* Radiofrequency ablation in 447 complex unresectable liver tumors: lessons learned. *Ann Surg Oncol* 2003; **10**: 52–8.

52. Llovet JM, Vilana R, Bru C, *et al.* Barcelona Clinic Liver Cancer (BCLC) Group. Increased risk of tumor seeding after percutaneous radiofrequency ablation for single hepatocellular carcinoma. *Hepatology* 2001; **33**: 1124–9.

9

Radiofrequency equipment and scientific basis for radiofrequency ablation

Suvranu Ganguli and S. Nahum Goldberg

Introduction

Minimally invasive strategies for tumor ablation, such as radiofrequency (RF) thermal ablation, have now gained prominent attention for the focal destruction of hepatic malignancies and are considered mainline therapies for some focal malignancies [1–7]. Advantages of minimally invasive therapies compared to surgical resection include the anticipated reduction in morbidity and mortality, lower cost, the ability to perform procedures on outpatients, and the potential application in a wider spectrum of patients, including non-surgical candidates.

Thermal ablation strategies utilize alterations in tissue temperature to induce cellular disruption and tissue coagulation necrosis [1,3,5]. This chapter will provide a conceptual framework for the principles and theories that underlie focal thermal tumor therapy using radiofrequency ablation (RFA). Particular emphasis will be placed on design and current use of radiofrequency equipment. Furthermore, developing synergistic therapies that allow treatment design tailored to patient specific disease will be discussed, as it is anticipated that these will further increase long-term success rates.

Basic principles of radiofrequency ablation

Goals of minimally invasive tumor ablation

The ultimate strategy of RF thermal tumor ablation therapy for hepatic and other malignancies encompasses two specific objectives. First, through the application of energy, to attempt to completely eradicate all viable malignant cells within a designated area. Based upon studies examining tumor progression for patients undergoing surgical resection, and the demonstration of viable malignant cells

Interventional Radiological Treatment of Liver Tumors, ed. Andy Adam and Peter R. Mueller.
Published by Cambridge University Press. © Cambridge University Press 2009.

beyond visible tumor boundaries, tumor ablation therapies attempt to include at least a 1.0 cm "ablative" margin of seemingly normal tissue for liver, but less may be needed for some tumors such as kidney [3]. Secondly, while complete tumor eradication is of primary importance, specificity and accuracy of therapy is also required. One significant advantage of RF thermal ablation over conventional standard surgical resection is the potential minimal amount of normal tissue loss that occurs. For example, in primary liver tumors, where functional hepatic reserve is a primary predictive factor in long-term patient survival outcomes, image-guided tumor ablation therapies have documented success in minimizing iatrogenic damage to cirrhotic parenchyma surrounding focal malignancies [8,9]. This is also useful in other clinical instances such as the need for nephron-sparing treatments in patients with von Hippel–Lindau that are prone to the development of multiple renal cell carcinomas [10].

Multiple energy sources have been used to provide the energy necessary to induce coagulation necrosis. This focal energy deposition is primarily achieved through the placement of applicators in the center of a tumor, around which heating occurs. Hyperthermic (> 50 °C) ablation therapies include using RF and microwave (electromagnetic), laser (light), and ultrasound energy to generate focal increases in tissue temperature. Cryoablation has also been used for focal tissue destruction by alternating between sessions of freezing and thawing. Currently, the greatest number of clinical and experimental studies has been performed using RF-based ablative devices, and our review of the basic principles of hyperthermic ablative therapy will use RF as a representative model.

Radiofrequency induction of coagulation necrosis

Thermal strategies for ablation attempt to destroy tumor tissue in a minimally invasive manner while limiting injury to nearby structures [3,5,11,12]. Cosman *et al.* have shown that the resistive heating produced by RFA techniques leads to heat-based cellular death via thermal coagulation necrosis [13]. The amount of tumor destruction is determined by generated temperatures and their pattern of distribution within treated tissues.

Cellular homeostatic mechanisms can accommodate slight increases in temperature (to 40 °C). Although increased susceptibility to damage by other mechanisms (radiation, chemotherapy) is seen at hyperthermic temperatures between 42 and 45 °C, cell function and tumor growth continues even after prolonged exposure [14,15]. Irreversible cellular injury occurs when cells are heated to 46 °C for 60 minutes, and occurs more rapidly as the temperature rises [16]. Immediate cellular damage centers on protein coagulation of cytosolic and mitochondrial enzymes and nucleic acid–histone protein complexes [17,19]. This damage triggers cellular death over the course of several days. "Coagulation necrosis" is used to describe this thermal damage, even though ultimate manifestations of cell death may not fulfill strict histopathologic criteria of coagulative necrosis. This has implications with regard to clinical practice, as percutaneous biopsy and histopathologic interpretation may not be a reliable measure of adequate ablation. Optimal temperatures for ablation range from 50 to 100 °C. Extremely high temperatures (> 105 °C) result in tissue vaporization, which in turn impedes the flow of current and restricts total energy deposition [20].

However, the exact temperature at which cell death occurs is multifactorial and tissue-specific. Studies have shown that depending on heating time and the tissue being heated, maximum temperatures at the edge of the ablation range in value. Maximum temperatures at the edge of the ablation zone, known as the "critical temperature," have been shown to range from 30 °C to 77 °C for normal tissues and from 41 °C to 64 °C for tumor models (a 23 °C difference). Likewise, the total amount of heat administered for a given time, known as the thermal dose, varies significantly between different tissues [21]. Thus, the 50 °C isotherm can really only be used as a general guideline.

Radiofrequency ablation techniques and equipment

Principles of the bioheat equation

Success of thermal ablative strategies is contingent upon adequate heat delivery. The ability to heat large volumes of tissue in different environments is dependent on several factors encompassing both RF delivery and local physiological tissue characteristics. Pennes first described the relationship between this set of parameters as the bioheat equation [22]:

$$\rho_t c_t \partial T(r, t)/\partial t = \nabla(k_t \nabla T) - c_b \rho_b \; m \; \rho_t(T - T_b) + Q_p(r, t) + Q_m(r, t)$$

where: ρ_t, ρ_b = density of tissue, blood (kg/m^3)

$\quad c_t, c_b$ = specific heat of tissue, blood (W s kg^{-1} °C)

$\quad\quad k_t$ = thermal conductivity of tissue

$\quad\quad m$ = perfusion (blood flow rate per unit mass tissue) (m^3 kg^{-1} s)

$\quad\quad Q_p$ = power absorbed per unit volume of tissue

$\quad\quad Q_m$ = metabolic heating per unit volume of tissue

This equation was further simplified to a first approximation [5] to describe the basic relationship guiding thermal ablation induced coagulation necrosis as:

coagulation necrosis = (energy deposited × local tissue interactions) − heat loss.

Based on this equation, several strategies have been pursued and equipment has been designed to increase the amount of coagulation necrosis by improving tissue–energy interactions during thermal ablation. These strategies have centered on altering one of the three parameters of the simplified bioheat equation – increasing RF energy deposition, modulating tissue characteristics, or modifying tissue blood flow. Again, although this is a useful framework, it should be kept in mind that the absolute temperature achieved at any point within a tumor does not mean definitively that ablation has occurred, as the exact temperature at which cell death occurs is multifactorial and tissue-specific.

Creating clinically meaningful volumes of ablation

Complete and adequate destruction by RFA requires that the entire tumor (and usually an ablative margin) be subjected to cytotoxic temperatures. RF delivers a high-frequency (460–500 kHz) alternating current into the tumor by means of an RF electrode, a thin needle (usually 21–14 gauge) or a set of needles that is electrically insulated along all but the distal 1–3 cm of the shaft. The application of RF current produces resistive friction in the tissue that is converted into heat [13]. Enhancement of the electrode design has played an essential role in achieving acceptable tissue tumor coagulation. Note that many of these ideas can and have been applied to other energy sources.

Modification of electrode design

Multitine arrays
Multitined expandable RF electrodes have been designed, with the deployment of a varying number of thin, curved tines in the shape of an umbrella or more complex geometries from a central cannula [23,24]. This allows placement of multiple probes to create large, reproducible volumes of necrosis. Leveen et al., using a 12-hook array, were able to produce lesions measuring up to 3.5 cm in diameter in in-vivo porcine liver by administering increasing amounts of RF energy from a 50 W RF generator for 10 minutes [25]. High-power systems (up to 250 W) have been developed with complex multitine electrode geometries and coagulations up

to 3.5 cm in diameter [26,27]. Subsequently, Berber *et al.* [28] have utilized multi-tine array systems to create reproducible ablation zones of more than 5 cm in diameter.

Bipolar/multipolar arrays

Several groups have worked with bipolar arrays instead of the conventional mono-polar system to increase the volume of coagulation. In these systems, applied RF current runs from an active electrode to a second grounding electrode in place of a grounding pad. Heat is generated around both electrodes, creating elliptical zones of coagulation. Desinger *et al.* described a bipolar array that contains both active and return electrodes on the same 2 mm diameter probe [29]. This arrangement eliminates the need for surface grounding pads and the risk of grounding-pad burns. Haemmerich *et al.* [30,31] further reported two multitined electrodes acting as both active and return to increase coagulation during bipolar RFA using a switching technique between electrodes to increase ablation efficiency. Lastly, multipolar devices that switch activation among a battery of bipolar electrodes are being used clinically, with promising results [32,33].

Internally cooled electrodes

One limitation to greater RF energy deposition has been overheating the tissues surrounding the active electrode, leading to tissue charring, rising impedance, and RF circuit interruption. To address this, internally cooled electrodes have been developed that are capable of greater coagulation compared to conventional mono-polar RF electrodes. These electrodes contain two hollow lumens that permit continuous internal cooling of the tip with a chilled perfusate and the removal of warmed effluent to a collection unit outside the body. This reduces heating directly around the electrode, minimizing tissue charring and rising impedance, allowing for greater RF energy deposition. Based upon success in inducing greater volumes of necrosis by using both multiprobe arrays and cooling, experiments have been performed with good results to study the use of internally cooled electrodes in clusters and in array [34,35].

Perfused electrodes

Perfusion electrodes have also been developed. These have small apertures at the active tip, allowing fluids (normal or hypertonic saline) to be infused or injected into the tissue before, during, or after the ablation procedure. The hypotheses for improved coagulation using these devices include effectively increasing the area of the active surface electrode from high-ion surrounding fluid, reduced effects of tissue vaporization (i.e., allowing probe–tissue contact despite the formation of electrically insulating gases), or improved thermal conduction caused by diffusion of boiling solution into the tissues.

Curley and Hamilton [36] infused up to 10 ml per min of normal saline in ex-vivo liver during RF application, and Livraghi *et al.* [37] reported using continuous infusion of normal saline at 1 ml per min in experimental animal models and human liver tumors. Novel "cooled-wet" techniques have been used to significantly increase RF-induced coagulation using a continuous saline infusion combined with an expandable electrode system [38–40].

RF algorithms for effective heating

Energy-deposition algorithms have been developed in an attempt to further improve heating over the volume of the tissue. For example, when pulsing is used, periods of high energy deposition are rapidly alternated with periods of low energy deposition. Preferential tissue cooling occurs adjacent to the electrode during periods of minimal energy deposition without significantly decreasing heating deeper in the tissue. Thus even greater energy can be applied during periods of high energy deposition, thereby enabling deeper heat penetration and greater tissue coagulation [34]. Each manufacturer has developed unique energy-deposition algorithms including pulsed energy (Valley Lab, Boulder, CO, USA), ramped increases in current (Boston Scientific, Natick, MA, USA), and stepped tine deployment (RITA Medical Systems, Fremont, CA, USA). Likewise, the end point for power deposition for each system is different, including time (Valley Lab), rising impedance (Boston Scientific), and temperature (RITA). Most likely, a combination of these algorithms will be found to be most effective in the future.

Modulating tissue characteristics

While modifications in electrode design and application protocols have yielded significant increases in coagulation volume compared to conventional monopolar RF systems, RF equipment modifications have not produced equivalent increases in clinical settings. This is largely due to multiple and often tissue-specific limitations that prevent heating of the entire tumor volume [12,20]. Most important is the heterogeneity of heat deposition throughout a given tumor to be treated. Recent attention has centered on altering underlying tumor physiology as a means to advance RF thermal ablation. Modifications of local tissue characteristics can be defined by changes in the thermal and electrical conductivity of the surrounding tissue.

Altered tissue thermal conductivity

As discussed for perfusion electrodes, improved heat conduction within the tissues by injection of saline and other compounds has been proposed [36,38,39,41]. The heated liquid spreads thermal energy farther and faster than heat conduction in normal "solid" tissue. An additional potential benefit of simultaneous saline injection is increased tissue ionicity, thereby enabling greater flow of current, as described below. Using ex-vivo agar phantoms and computer modeling, lower thermal conductivity of background tissues has been shown to significantly increase temperatures within a defined ablation target [42]. These findings provide insight into the "oven effect" (i.e., increased heating efficacy for tumors surrounded by cirrhotic liver or fat, such as exophytic renal cell carcinomas) and highlight the importance of both the tumor and the surrounding tissue characteristics when contemplating ablation efficacy.

Altered tissue electrical conductivity

For a given RF current, the power deposition at each point in space is strongly dependent on the local electrical conductivity. We and other investigators have demonstrated the ability to increase coagulation volume by altering electrical conductivity in tissues through saline injection prior to or during RF ablation [43,44]. In general, small volumes of highly concentrated sodium ions are injected in and around the ablation site to maximize local heating effects rather than global heating effects [43]. Using perfused electrodes with saline may require higher power generators; however, using this technique can heat deeper into tissues than is achieved without saline treatments [43,44].

Modulating tissue blood flow

The foremost factor limiting thermal ablation of tumors in in-vivo settings continues to be tissue blood flow [45]. RFA outcomes in in-vivo models have been less successful and more variable than reported reproducible ex-vivo results for identical RF protocols. RF-induced necrosis in vivo is often shaped by the presence of vasculature in the vicinity of the ablation. This reduced RF coagulation necrosis in in-vivo settings is a result of both visible vessels and perfusion-mediated tissue cooling (capillary vascular flow), which functions as a heat sink. By drawing heat from the treatment zone, this effect reduces the volume of tissue that receives the required minimal thermal dose for coagulation. Several studies exploring altered tissue perfusion and the heat-sink effect to increase the ablative zone through either mechanical occlusion or pharmacologic agents strongly support the contention that perfusion-mediated tissue cooling is responsible for this reduction in observed coagulation.

Minimizing heat sink

Mechanical occlusion. In a study in an in-vivo porcine model, Lu *et al.* examined the effect of hepatic vessel diameter on RFA outcome [46]. Using CT and histopathologic analysis, more complete thermal heating and a reduced heat-sink effect was identified when hepatic vessels within the heating zone were < 3mm in diameter. In contrast, vessels > 3mm in diameter had higher patency rates, less endothelial injury, and greater viability of surrounding hepatocytes after RFA. This strong predictive nature of hepatic blood flow on the extent of RF-induced coagulation has been confirmed in multiple studies where increased coagulation volumes have been obtained when hepatic blood flow is decreased, either by balloon or coil embolization or by the Pringle maneuver [47–49].

Tissue perfusion

Pharmacologic modulation of blood flow. Pharmacologic modulation of blood flow and anti-angiogenesis therapy are promising techniques. Goldberg *et al.* modulated hepatic blood flow using intra-arterial vasopressin and high-dose halothane in conjunction with RFA in in-vivo porcine liver [50]. Arsenic trioxide has received increasing attention as a novel anti-neoplastic agent [51]. In a renal tumor model in rabbits, Horkan *et al.* [52] showed that arsenic trioxide preferentially decreased tumor blood flow and significantly increased RF-induced coagulation. Promising anti-angiogenic therapies, such as sorafenib [53], are also starting to be studied in combination therapies.

Synergistic therapies

Given the high likelihood of incomplete treatment by heat-based modalities alone, especially for tumors larger than 3–5 cm, treatments combining thermal ablation with therapies such as radiation therapy, chemotherapy, and chemoembolization are being investigated and have shown substantial promise.

Thermal ablation with chemotherapy

Cellular hypoxic insults on tumor cells caused by prior tumor cell damage from chemotherapy (adjuvant) can be used to increase tumor sensitivity to heat [54,55]. Alternatively, tumor cells undergoing heat-induced reversible cell injury may demonstrate increased susceptibility to secondary chemotherapy. Synergy between chemotherapy and hyperthermic temperatures (42–45 °C) has already been well established [15,56], and the combination and optimization of thermal ablation and chemotherapy is a key direction for further research. Along these lines, several animal studies and at least one clinical study combining RFA with liposomal doxorubicin demonstrated increases in coagulation and reduced tumor growth rates over either therapy alone [57–59].

Several papers have described RF ablation combined with percutaneous alcohol injection [60,61] and transhepatic arterial chemoembolization [62]. For example, Kitamoto *et al.* [62] treated a series of 26 nodules of hepatocellular carcinoma in 21 patients. All nodules underwent RF ablation and 10 nodules non-randomly selected underwent transhepatic arterial chemoembolization with doxorubicin–lipiodol at some point (average 18.2 days) prior to RFA. The authors concluded that the combination of RFA and transhepatic arterial chemoembolization markedly increased the extent of induced coagulation compared with RFA alone and decreased the amount of local tumor recurrence. These combination therapies are another area of potential combination tumor therapy that will receive greater attention in the near future.

Thermal ablation with radiation therapy

Recently, investigators have begun exploring combination RFA and radiation therapy, with promising results. Previous data in the literature have demonstrated increased tumor destruction with external-beam radiation therapy and low-temperature hyperthermia [63,66]. Potential causes for the synergy between hyperthermia and radiation therapy include increased oxygenation in blood flow to the tumor, caused by local hyperthermia induced in tissues peripheral to the ablated region. Increased oxygenation has been implicated in the sensitization of the tumor to subsequent radiation therapy [67]. Another possible mechanism, which has been seen in animal tumor models, is an inhibition of radiation-induced repair and recovery and increased free radical formation [68]. Future work is needed to identify the optimal temperature for ablation and optimal radiation dose, as well as the most effective method of administering radiation therapy (external-beam radiation therapy vs. brachytherapy or yttrium microspheres), on an organ-by-organ basis [69].

Conclusion

Minimally invasive radiofrequency ablation has been well described for use in the treatment of focal hepatic malignancies. Investigators have characterized many of the basic principles underlying the tumor ablative features of this treatment. We have provided an overview of the basic principles of RFA and described the equipment and technologic modifications that have been developed to further improve clinical success of this therapy. Future research is now looking to combination therapies as a means of further improving clinical effectiveness.

REFERENCES

1. Ahmed M, Goldberg SN. Thermal ablation therapy for hepatocellular carcinoma. *J Vasc Interv Radiol* 2002; **13** (9 Suppl): S231–44.
2. Colella G, Bottelli R, De Carlis L, *et al.* Hepatocellular carcinoma: comparison between liver transplantation, resective surgery, ethanol injection, and chemoembolization. *Transpl Int* 1998; **11** (Suppl 1): S193–6.
3. Dodd GD 3rd, Soulen MC, Kane RA, *et al.* Minimally invasive treatment of malignant hepatic tumors: at the threshold of a major breakthrough. *Radiographics* 2000; **20**: 9–27.
4. Goldberg SN, Dupuy DE. Image-guided radiofrequency tumor ablation: challenges and opportunities. Part I. *J Vasc Interv Radiol* 2001; **12**: 1021–32.
5. Goldberg SN, Gazelle GS, Mueller PR. Thermal ablation therapy for focal malignancy: a unified approach to underlying principles, techniques, and diagnostic imaging guidance. *AJR Am J Roentgenol* 2000; **174**: 323–31.
6. Giorgio A, Tarantino L, de Stefano G, Coppola C, Ferraioli G. Complications after percutaneous saline-enhanced radiofrequency ablation of liver tumors: 3-year experience with 336 patients at a single center. *AJR Am J Roentgenol* 2005; **184**: 207–11.
7. Livraghi T, Solbiati L, Meloni MF, *et al.* Treatment of focal liver tumors with percutaneous radio-frequency ablation: complications encountered in a multicenter study. *Radiology* 2003; **226**: 441–51.
8. Lencioni R, Cioni D, Crocetti L, *et al.* Early-stage hepatocellular carcinoma in patients with cirrhosis: long-term results of percutaneous image-guided radiofrequency ablation. *Radiology* 2005; **234**: 961–7.

9. Kim YK, Kim CS, Chung GH, *et al.* Radiofrequency ablation of hepatocellular carcinoma in patients with decompensated cirrhosis: evaluation of therapeutic efficacy and safety. *AJR Am J Roentgenol* 2006; **186** (5 Suppl): S261–8.

10. Clark TW, Millward SF, Gervais DA, *et al.* Reporting standards for percutaneous thermal ablation of renal cell carcinoma. *J Vasc Interv Radiol* 2006; **17**: 1563–70.

11. Gazelle GS, Goldberg SN, Solbiati L, Livraghi T. Tumor ablation with radiofrequency energy. *Radiology* 2000; **217**: 6333–46.

12. McGahan JP, Dodd GD 3rd. Radiofrequency ablation of the liver: current status. *AJR Am J Roentgenol* 2001; **176**: 3–16.

13. Cosman E, Nashold B, Ovelman-Levitt J. Theoretical aspects of radiofrequency lesions in the dorsal root entry zone. *Neurosurgery* 1984; **15**: 945–50.

14. Seegenschmiedt M, Brady L, Sauer R. Interstitial thermoradiotherapy: review on technical and clinical aspects. *Am J Clin Oncol* 1990; **13**: 352–63.

15. Trembley B, Ryan T, Strohbehn J. Interstitial hyperthermia: physics, biology, and clinical aspects. In: *Hyperthermia and Oncology*, Vol. 3. Utrecht: VSP, 1992: 11–98.

16. Larson T, Bostwick D, Corcia A. Temperature-correlated histopathologic changes following microwave thermoablation of obstructive tissues in patients with benign prostatic hyperplasia. *Urology* 1996; **47**: 463–9.

17. Zevas N, Kuwayama A. Pathologic analysis of experimental thermal lesions: comparison of induction heating and radiofrequency electrocoagulation. *J Neurosurg* 1972; **37**: 418–22.

18. Thomsen S. Pathologic analysis of photothermal and photomechanical effects of laser tissue interactions. *Photochem Photobiol* 1991; **53**: 825–35.

19. Goldberg SN, Gazelle GS, Compton CC, Mueller PR, Tanabe KK. Treatment of intrahepatic malignancy with radiofrequency ablation: radiologic–pathologic correlation. *Cancer* 2000; **88**: 2452–63.

20. Goldberg SN, Gazelle GS, Halpern EF, *et al.* Radiofrequency tissue ablation: importance of local temperature along the electrode tip exposure in determining lesion shape and size. *Acad Radiol* 1996; **3**: 212–8.

21. Liu Z, Lobo SM, Humphries S, *et al.* Radiofrequency tumor ablation: insight into improved efficacy using computer modeling. *AJR Am J Roentgenol* 2005; **184**: 1347–52.

22. Pennes HH. Analysis of tissue and arterial blood temperatures in the resting human forearm. *J Appl Physiol* 1948; **1**: 93–122.

23. Rossi S, Buscarini E, Garbagnati F. Percutaneous treatment of small hepatic tumors by an expandable RF needle electrode. *AJR Am J Roentgenol* 1998; **170**: 1015–22.

24. Siperstein AE, Rogers SJ, Hansen PD, Gitomirsky A. Laparoscopic thermal ablation of hepatic neuroendocrine tumor metastases. *Surgery* 1997; **122**: 1147–55.

25. Leveen RF. Laser hyperthermia and radiofrequency ablation of hepatic lesions. *Semin Interv Radiol* 1997; **12**: 313–24.

26. Berber E, Foroutani A, Garland AM, *et al.* Use of CT Hounsfield unit density to identify ablated tumor after laparoscopic radiofrequency ablation of hepatic tumors. *Surg Endosc* 2000; **14**: 799–804.

27. de Baere T, Denys A, Wood BJ, *et al.* Radiofrequency liver ablation: experimental comparative study of water-cooled versus expandable systems. *AJR Am J Roentgenol* 2001; **176**: 187–92.

28. Berber E, Herceg NL, Casto KJ, Siperstein AE. Laparoscopic radiofrequency ablation of hepatic tumors: prospective clinical evaluation of ablation size comparing two treatment algorithms. *Surg Endosc* 2004; **18**: 390–6.

29. Desinger K, Stein T, Muller G, Mack M, Vogl T. Interstitial bipolar RF-thermotherapy (REITT) therapy planning by computer simulation and MRI-monitoring: a new concept for minimally invasive procedures. *Proc SPIE* 1999; **3249**: 147–60.

30. Haemmerich DG, Lee FT, Chachati L, *et al.* A device that allows for multiple simultaneous radiofrequency (RF) ablations in separated areas of the liver with impedance-controlled cool-ip probes: an ex vivo feasibility study. *Radiology* 2002; **225**(p): 242.

31. Haemmerich DG, Lee FT, Mahvi DM, Wright AS, Webster JG. Multiple probe radiofrequency: rapid switching versus simultaneous power application in a computer model. *Radiology* 2002; **225**(p): 639.

32. Terraz S, Constantin C, Majno PE, *et al.* Image-guided multipolar radiofrequency ablation of liver tumours: initial clinical results. *Eur Radiol* 2007; **17**: 2253–61.

33. Clasen S, Schmidt D, Boss A, *et al.* Multipolar radiofrequency ablation with internally cooled electrodes: experimental study in ex vivo bovine liver with mathematic modeling. *Radiology* 2006; **238**: 881–90.

34. Goldberg SN, Solbiati L, Hahn PF, *et al.* Large-volume tissue ablation with radio frequency by using a clustered, internally cooled electrode technique: laboratory and clinical experience in liver metastases. *Radiology* 1998; **209**: 371–9.

35. Hines-Peralta A, Liu ZJ, Horkan C, Solazzo S, Goldberg SN. Chemical tumor ablation with use of a novel multiple-tine infusion system in a canine sarcoma model. *J Vasc Interv Radiol* 2006; **17**: 351–8.

36. Curley MG, Hamilton PS. Creation of large thermal lesions in liver using saline-enhanced RF ablation. *Proc 19th International Conference IEEE/EMBS* 1997: 2516–9.

37. Livraghi T, Goldberg SN, Monti F, *et al.* Saline-enhanced radiofrequency tissue ablation in the treatment of liver metastases. *Radiology* 1997; **202**: 205–10.

38. Miao Y, Ni Y, Yu J, Marchal G. A comparative study on validation of a novel cooled-wet electrode for radiofrequency liver ablation. *Invest Radiol* 2000; **35**: 438–44.

39. Miao Y, Ni Y, Yu J, Zhang H, Baert A, Marchal G. An ex vivo study on radiofrequency tissue ablation: increased lesion size by using an "expandable-wet" electrode. *Eur Radiol* 2001; **11**: 1841–7.

40. Kettenbach J, Kostler W, Rucklinger E, *et al.* Percutaneous saline-enhanced radiofrequency ablation of unresectable liver tumors: initial experience in 26 patients. *AJR Am J Roentgenol* 2003; **180**: 1537–45.

41. Leveillee RJ, Hoey MF. Radiofrequency interstitial tissue ablation: wet electrode. *J Endourol* 2003; **17**: 563–77.

42. Liu Z, Ahmed M, Weinstein Y, *et al.* Characterization of the RF ablation-induced "oven effect": the importance of background tissue thermal conductivity on tissue heating. *Int J Hyperthermia* 2006; **22**: 327–42.

43. Aube C, Schmidt D, Brieger J, *et al.* Influence of NaCl concentrations on coagulation, temperature, and electrical conductivity using a perfusion radiofrequency ablation system: an ex vivo experimental study. *Cardiovasc Intervent Radiol* 2007; **30**: 92–7.

44. Lobo SM, Afzal KS, Ahmed M, *et al.* Radiofrequency ablation: modeling the enhanced temperature response to adjuvant NaCl pretreatment. *Radiology* 2004; **230**: 175–82.

45. Brown DB. Concepts, considerations, and concerns on the cutting edge of radiofrequency ablation. *J Vasc Interv Radiol* 2005; **16**: 597–613.

46. Lu DS, Raman SS, Vodopich DJ, *et al.* Effect of vessel size on creation of hepatic radiofrequency lesions in pigs: assessment of the "heat sink" effect. *AJR Am J Roentgenol* 2002; **178**: 47–51.

47. Patterson EJ, Scudamore CH, Owen DA, Nagy AG, Buczkowski AK. Radiofrequency ablation of porcine liver in vivo: effects of blood flow and treatment time on lesion size. *Ann Surg* 1998; **227**: 559–65.

48. Frich L, Mala T, Gladhaug IP. Hepatic radiofrequency ablation using perfusion electrodes in a pig model: effect of the Pringle manoeuvre. *Eur J Surg Oncol* 2006; **32**: 527–32.

49. Chinn SB, Lee FT Jr, Kennedy GD, *et al.* Effect of vascular occlusion on radiofrequency ablation of the liver: results in a porcine model. *AJR Am J Roentgenol* 2001; **176**: 789–95.

50. Goldberg SN, Hahn PF, Halpern EF, Fogle R, Gazelle GS. Radiofrequency tissue ablation: effect of pharmacologic modulation of blood flow on coagulation diameter. *Radiology* 1998; **209**: 761–9.

51. Murgo AJ. Clinical trials of arsenic trioxide in hematologic and solid tumors: overview of the National Cancer Institute Cooperative Research and Development Studies. *Oncologist* 2001; **6** (Suppl 2): 22–8.

52. Horkan C, Ahmed M, Liu Z, *et al.* Radiofrequency ablation: effect of pharmacologic modulation of hepatic and renal blood flow on coagulation diameter in a VX2 tumor model. *J Vasc Interv Radiol* 2004; **15**: 269–74.

53. Ratain MJ, Eisen T, Stadler WM, *et al.* Phase II placebo-controlled randomized discontinuation trial of sorafenib in patients with metastatic renal cell carcinoma. *J Clin Oncol* 2006; **24**: 2505–12.

54. Pautler SE, Pavlovich CP, Mikityansky I, *et al.* Retroperitoneoscopic-guided radiofrequency ablation of renal tumors. *Can J Urol* 2001; **8**: 1330–3.

55. Pavlovich CP, Walther MM, Choyke PL, *et al.* Percutaneous radio frequency ablation of small renal tumors: initial results. *J Urol* 2002; **167**: 10–15.

56. Christophi C, Muralidharan V. Treatment of hepatocellular carcinoma by percutaneous laser hyperthermia. *J Gastroenterol Hepatol* 2001; **16**: 548–52.

57. Ahmed M, Liu Z, Lukyanov AN, *et al.* Combination radiofrequency ablation with intratumoral liposomal doxorubicin: effect on drug accumulation and coagulation in multiple tissues and tumor types in animals. *Radiology* 2005; **235**: 469–77.

58. Ahmed M, Lukyanov AN, Torchilin V, *et al.* Combined radiofrequency ablation and adjuvant liposomal chemotherapy: effect of chemotherapeutic agent, nanoparticle size, and circulation time. *J Vasc Interv Radiol* 2005; **16**: 1365–71.

59. Goldberg SN, Kamel IR, Kruskal JB, *et al.* Radiofrequency ablation of hepatic tumors: increased tumor destruction with adjuvant liposomal doxorubicin therapy. *AJR Am J Roentgenol* 2002; **179**: 93–101.

60. Watanabe S, Kurokohchi K, Masaki T, *et al.* Enlargement of thermal ablation zone by the combination of ethanol injection and radiofrequency ablation in excised bovine liver. *Int J Oncol* 2004; **24**: 279–84.

61. Kurokohchi K, Watanabe S, Masaki T, *et al.* Comparison between combination therapy of percutaneous ethanol injection and radiofrequency ablation and radiofrequency ablation alone for patients with hepatocellular carcinoma. *World J Gastroenterol* 2005; **11**: 1426–32.

62. Kitamoto M, Imagawa M, Yamada H, *et al.* Radiofrequency ablation in the treatment of small hepatocellular carcinomas: comparison of the radiofrequency effect with and without chemoembolization. *AJR Am J Roentgenol* 2003; **181**: 997–1003.

63. Xia T, Sun Q, Shi X, Fan N, Hiraoka M. Relationship between thermal parameters and tumor response in hyperthermia combined with radiation therapy. *Int J Clin Oncol* 2001; **6**: 138–42.

64. Kalapurakal JA, Pierce M, Chen A, Sathiaseelan V. Efficacy of irradiation and external hyperthermia in locally advanced, hormone-refractory or radiation recurrent prostate cancer: a preliminary report. *Int J Radiat Oncol Biol Phys* 2003; **57**: 654–64.

65. Sakurai H, Hayakawa K, Mitsuhashi N, *et al.* Effect of hyperthermia combined with external radiation therapy in primary non-small cell lung cancer with direct bony invasion. *Int J Hyperthermia* 2002; **18**: 472–83.

66. van der Zee J, Gonzalez Gonzalez D, van Rhoon GC, *et al.* Comparison of radiotherapy alone with radiotherapy plus hyperthermia in locally advanced pelvic tumours: a prospective, randomised, multicentre trial. Dutch Deep Hyperthermia Group. *Lancet* 2000; **355**: 1119–25.

67. Horkan C, Dalal K, Coderre JA, *et al.* Reduced tumor growth with combined radiofrequency ablation and radiation therapy in a rat breast tumor model. *Radiology* 2005; **235**: 81–8.

68. Rhamanuddin S, Solazzo S, Mahadevan A, *et al.* Combined radiofrequency (RF) thermal ablation and radiation therapy (XRT) increases parameters indicative of oxidative and nitrosative stress as well as increasing tumor coagulation. *Annual Meeting of the Radiological Society of North America*, Chicago, 2007.

69. Dupuy DE, DiPetrillo T, Gandhi S, *et al.* Radiofrequency ablation followed by conventional radiotherapy for medically inoperable stage I non-small cell lung cancer. *Chest* 2006; **129**: 738–45.

10

Cryotherapy of the liver

Gregory Avey, Fred T. Lee Jr., and J. Louis Hinshaw

Introduction

For the purposes of cryoablation planning, hepatic malignancies can be divided into primary hepatic neoplasms and metastatic disease. While the performance of the cryoablation procedure is similar for both primary and metastatic lesions, patient selection and follow-up is very different. In both cases, proper patient selection and treatment ideally involves a multidisciplinary team with skills in systemic chemotherapy, embolization, internal radiation, surgery, ablation, transplantation, and supportive care, as appropriate, to optimize the patient's treatment.

Hepatocellular carcinoma (HCC) accounts for the majority of primary hepatic malignancies, and also the corresponding bulk of ablations for primary liver masses. The incidence of hepatocellular carcinoma has been steadily rising due to the increase in hepatitis B and C, and the affected patient population is becoming younger [1,2]. In the setting of chronic viral hepatitis and subsequent cirrhosis, there is a strong "field effect" on susceptible liver tissue that places the patient at risk for developing hepatocellular carcinoma as well as synchronous and metachronous sites of disease [3].

Colon cancer is the most common metastatic liver lesion. Because of the pattern of portal blood flow, the liver is often the initial and sometimes the only site of metastasis. While other primary cancers such as melanoma, carcinoid, renal cell carcinoma, and pancreatic neoplasms metastasize to the liver, these tumors are highly associated with systemic spread, making locoregional therapies less effective [4]. Therefore, this discussion of the cryoablation of metastatic lesions will concentrate on colorectal cancer, although there may be indications for ablation in individual cases of other metastatic malignancies.

The US National Cancer Institute estimated that 153 760 men and women would be diagnosed with colon and rectal cancer in 2007, with more than 50 000 deaths [5].

Interventional Radiological Treatment of Liver Tumors, ed. Andy Adam and Peter R. Mueller.
Published by Cambridge University Press. © Cambridge University Press 2009.

Most of the patients that succumb to colon cancer have hepatic metastatic disease at the time of death. Unfortunately, only about 25% of patients with hepatic metastatic disease are candidates for surgical resection [6]. Cryoablation provides another treatment option for those patients who are unable to tolerate resection. Hepatic cryoablation is a focal ablative technique, which has been used as an adjunct to resection for many years. In other patients with limited disease not amenable to resection, or in patients whose condition precludes resection, cryoablation can be used with curative intent.

Tissue freezing during cryoablation causes both intracellular and extracellular formation of ice. The location of ice formation and therefore mechanism of cell death varies with the rate and final temperature of freezing. Freezing at faster rates and to lower temperatures promotes the formation of intracellular ice crystals. Intracellular ice crystals cause cell death though direct damage to the cell membrane and organelles. Conversely, slower rates of freezing favor the formation of extra-cellular ice crystals. The extracellular ice-crystal formation leaves the remainder of the extracellular milieu relatively hyperosmolar to the intracellular compartment, thereby leading to cell dehydration and death [7].

The temperature necessary to cause reliable cellular necrosis depends on both cell and tissue type. Some investigators have demonstrated that individual cell lines may remain viable despite freezing to −35 °C [8]. However, in-vivo testing in water-rich tumors demonstrates reliable zones of necrosis in regions near the periphery of the cryoablation zone (at approximately the −20 °C isotherm), an effect attributed to the formation of extracellular ice in the hepatic sinusoids and disruption of the hepatic microvasculature [9]. More fibrous tumors may require temperatures as low as −40 °C, an isotherm that is typically achieved 8 mm within the iceball as visualized on imaging [10].

Work-up and patient selection

Hepatocellular carcinoma

As discussed previously, the incidence of HCC has been increasing and the average age of onset has been decreasing, trends which have been attributed to the increasing prevalence of hepatitis B and C [1]. HCC almost exclusively arises in the setting of chronic liver injury with associated cirrhosis. By the time HCC presents symptomatically, it is often advanced, limiting the utility of local treatment options. Given these factors, an adequate screening program of patients with cirrhosis is vital to detect HCC at the stage of localized disease amenable to ablation therapy. In patients with risk factors for the development of HCC, annual or biannual screening exams in conjunction with measurement of serum alpha-fetoprotein has been shown to decrease mortality and improve early detection of tumor [11]. While screening is an imperfect practice, recent reviews have found that screening with ultrasound (US), computed tomography (CT), and magnetic resonance imaging (MRI) provides estimated sensitivities ranging from 60% to 81% and specificities ranging from 85% to 97% [12].

The preferred treatment in patients with limited disease is hepatic transplant (when feasible), and the next most effective treatment is hepatic resection [13,14]. However, orthotopic liver transplant is a limited resource largely confined to wealthy countries with well-developed healthcare systems. Due to the limited utilization of screening and the aggressive nature of HCC, only 20–30% of patients are eligible for surgical resection at the time of diagnosis [15]. Patients may be excluded from resection due to limited hepatic reserve, proximity of the tumor to major intrahepatic vessels, or high surgical risk. In those for whom surgical therapy is contraindicated, treatment options include ablative therapies (thermal or chemical), embolization (bland, chemotherapeutic, and radioactive), and intra-arterial chemotherapy. Unfortunately, systemic chemotherapy has not been shown to be effective in the treatment of HCC, with the best therapy to date providing only a 3-month time-to-progression advantage [16]. Given the wide range of treatment options, the involvement of a multispeciality group is instrumental in achieving the best possible care for each patient.

HCC recurs frequently even if ablative therapies are provided with curative intent. Many series report a local recurrence rate ranging from 0% to 27% [17–19]. More commonly, however, patients present with metachronous lesions or intrahepatic metastasis [20]. The overall 3-year recurrence rate for surgical resection and for ablative therapies is approximately 50% [21].

Metastatic disease

Ablative therapies are more likely to be of benefit in patients with colorectal metastases than in those with metastases from other primary sites. The majority of patients with non-colorectal metastatic liver tumors usually have widespread micrometastatic deposits in the liver and metastases elsewhere in the body. In a small subset of patients with relatively indolent non-colorectal metastases such as breast cancer, indolent renal cell metastases, and neuroendocrine tumors, ablation has been shown to increase survival [22–24]. Ablation of these lesions should be considered based on the specifics of the individual case.

As with HCC, surgical resection is considered the optimal therapy in eligible patients with metastatic colorectal cancer. If resection is possible, several series have demonstrated mean 5-year survivals of 32–58% [25–28]. However, up to 80% of patients with colorectal cancer are not candidates for surgical resection at the time of presentation [29]. Median survival in this group of patients with unresectable hepatic disease is approximately 6 months without treatment [30,31]. Unlike in patients with HCC, systemic chemotherapy is effective in increasing mean survival in patients with metastatic colorectal cancer, with current chemotherapeutic regimens showing mean survival of approximately 16–20 months [32,33]. Recent studies have suggested that the addition of angiogenesis inhibitors may prolong mean survival beyond 24 months [34]. Given the success of the combination of surgical and chemotherapeutic options for the treatment of colorectal metastasis, ablative therapies are usually offered to patients who are not surgical candidates. Many patients are not resection candidates because of poor health, widespread tumor, metastases in those who have previously undergone resection, or tumors in locations not amenable to resection. In selected cases, a partial hepatectomy can be performed with accompanying ablation of isolated lesions in the remaining liver.

Studies have demonstrated that certain subgroups are at increased risk for developing recurrence despite adequate ablation. In one series, tumors greater than 3 cm in size were shown to be at significantly increased risk of local recurrence [17]. Additionally, those with serum levels of carcinoembryonic antigen (CEA) greater than 100 ng mL^{-1} preoperatively and 5 ng mL^{-1} postoperatively were shown to have shorter disease-free survival [35]. While an increase in the number of lesions has not been shown to increase the risk of recurrence [35], there is a practical limit to the number of lesions that may be treated in one setting. The typical limit at our center is five hepatic lesions, each less than 5 cm in size. This is based on data from the surgical literature, which suggests that metastasectomy is less effective with extensive metastatic disease, and the practical logistical aspects of ablating more numerous lesions. However, each case is independently reviewed, and in some cases this criterion is expanded. For example, more numerous and/or larger lesions may be targeted in a symptomatic patient with neuroendocrine tumor for tumor debulking and symptom-control purposes. Additional factors, such as coagulopathy or low hepatic functional reserve, are considerations, but seldom preclude indicated treatment. Ablative treatment is almost never indicated in patients with gross extrahepatic metastases.

Technique

The goal in cryoablation is to produce a zone of necrosis extending beyond the tumor to a suitable margin. While the technique of placing and monitoring the probes is similar for both HCC and colorectal metastases, the preferred margin and susceptibility to cryoablation is different. HCC, being a relatively water-rich tumor, is more susceptible to the effects of cryoablation than the more fibrous colorectal cancer metastases. Additionally, there is often greater need to preserve viable hepatic tissue in patients with HCC than in those with colorectal cancer. Therefore, while a surrounding 1 cm surgical margin is desirable when treating metastatic disease, a smaller margin is often used in patients with HCC [36].

Traditional cryoprobes achieved the freezing effect by circulating liquid nitrogen out to the tip of a metallic probe. However, the probes were too large to be safely placed percutaneously. More recently, probes have become available which operate on the Joule–Thompson principle of expanding gases. In these probes, argon gas is allowed to expand from a pressurized system into a decompression chamber, which results in cooling. This has allowed the manufacture of smaller cryoprobes between 13 and 17 gauge, thus enabling percutaneous placement. Both intraoperative and percutaneous systems allow simultaneous placement of multiple cryoprobes and provide continuous monitoring of the temperature of the iceball core. There are also MRI-compatible percutaneous cryoablation probes.

Probe placement

One of the major advantages of cryoablation is the ability to use numerous probes to ablate large and irregularly shaped lesions. Probes can also be placed in close proximity to vascular structures, and sometimes even freeze the vessels shut (Fig. 10.1). The "2–1" rule published by Wang et al. is a useful guide to planning probe placement [37]. The 2–1 rule states that cryoprobes should be placed no more than 1 cm from the lesion edge, and no farther than 2 cm from the nearest cryoprobe. As a result, this gives a 1 cm sphere of influence for each cryoprobe placed. Placement in this arrangement allows synergistic effects from cryoprobes, providing both a greater rate of freezing and a larger isotherm of temperatures less than −20 to −40 °C. These high rates of freezing and low temperatures have been shown to ensure cell death. While a 2 cm lesion could in theory be treated with placement of a single probe, the synergy of two cryoprobes favors the use of a minimum of two cryoprobes for lesions of this size. For lesions less than 2 cm in size, a single cryoprobe is often sufficient.

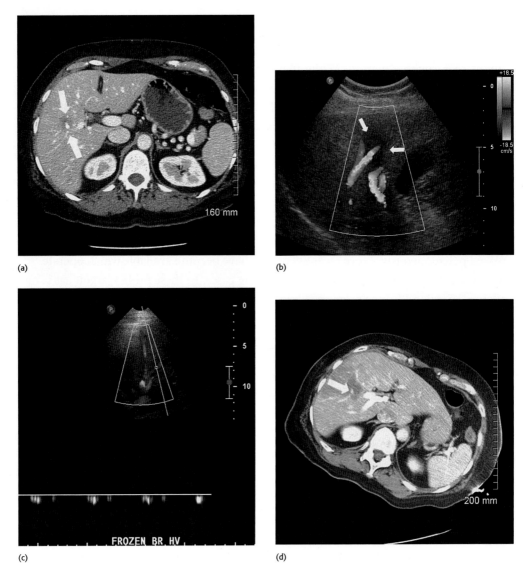

(a)

(b)

(c)

(d)

Figure 10.1 (a) Contrast-enhanced CT image through the abdomen in a patient with a history of metastatic breast cancer. There is a new hypoenhancing hepatic mass surrounding a relatively large (4 mm) branch of the middle hepatic vein (arrows). (b) Color Doppler image prior to cryoablation identifying brisk flow within the hepatic venous branch coursing through the hypoechoic lesion (arrows). (c) Color and pulsed Doppler image during cryoablation shows some probable transmitted pulsations, but no real flow within the more proximal hepatic venous branch after the iceball had enveloped the mass and hepatic vein. (d) Contrast-enhanced CT image through the abdomen following the cryoablation and thawing of the iceball. The hepatic venous branch has re-cannulated (arrow). *See color plate section.*

Vascular anatomy is also an important consideration when planning the placement of the cryoprobes. Large vascular structures can act as a "cold sink", with the blood flow dissipating some of the cooling potential. Larger vascular structures are unlikely to be injured during the procedure, due to their fibrous nature and muscular composition. At least one study has documented normal arterial smooth muscle function following exposure to liquid nitrogen [38]. Due to the decreased effective range of cryoprobes in the region of the cold-sink phenomenon, it is recommended that probes be placed only 5 mm inside the margin of the tumor adjacent to the vessel, and that cryoprobes be placed no more than 1 cm apart in this region. Some centers have also used temporary occlusion of the hepatic inflow or hepatic vein outflow to decrease hepatic blood flow and thereby to minimize the cold-sink effect. Taking this, as well as the relative precision of cryoablation, into consideration, cryoablation can be used to treat relatively central lesions.

The percutaneous placement of cryoprobes is performed utilizing essentially identical techniques to those employed in radiofrequency ablation (RFA) and hepatic biopsy. US, CT, and MRI can all be used to effectively guide placement of the probes. US has the advantage of allowing real-time monitoring of the probe trajectory and the target. Ultrasound also typically provides superior conspicuity of the target lesion when compared to non-contrast CT. A subcostal approach is preferred and is feasible for the majority of lesions. Some lesions high in the dome of the liver may require intercostal puncture, and this can be performed safely since US also allows for real-time monitoring of the aerated lung edge, thus permitting placement without a significant risk of subsequent pneumothorax. A "protective pleural effusion" can be created to protect the lung base from injury for difficult dome lesions [39]. Other investigators, prompted by the use of RFA for lung lesions, have reported transpulmonary placement of probes utilizing CT guidance. However, this method did require placement of a temporary chest tube due to pneumothorax in 28% of the study population [40].

Percutaneous probe placement has the advantages of low morbidity, shorter recovery period, and a relatively short hospital stay [41]. However, if the particular circumstances of a case require intraoperative ultrasound (IOUS) probe placement, or if cryoablation is being done in conjunction with partial hepatectomy, there are some advantages to the exposure afforded by laparotomy. A combination of direct visualization and tactile evaluation can be used to assist with probe placement. IOUS has also been shown to be more sensitive than CT and MRI for the detection of unexpected lesions, and can alter surgical management [42]. If

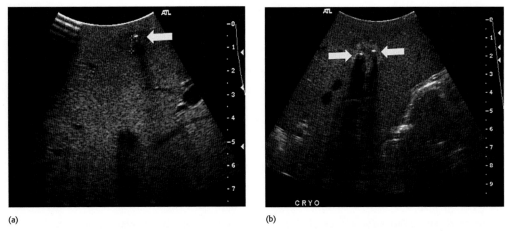

(a)   (b)

Figure 10.2 (a) Intraoperative US image during cryoprobe placement. The orientation of the probe is transverse to the orientation of the transducer. As a result, the probe appears as a hyperechoic focus on the US image (arrow). Multiple repositionings may be necessary to obtain optimal results since it can be difficult to estimate the correct depth and angle of the cryoprobe initially. (b) Intraoperative US image demonstrating the appearance of early iceball formation with hyperechoic foci developing around the cryoprobes, with associated posterior shadowing.

available, contrast-enhanced ultrasound has been demonstrated to be even more sensitive than CT, MRI, and IOUS in the detection of unexpected lesions, and in fact results in changes in surgical management in approximately 30% of the patients in whom it is used [43].

Cryoprobe placement with the intraoperative ultrasound transducer can be technically challenging, as conventional longitudinal images are difficult to obtain with the orientation of the IOUS transducer and cord. Placement of probes with oblique imaging may require multiple repositioning and placement verification, with associated prolongation of the procedure time (Fig. 10.2).

Monitoring of the ablation zone

Probably the most significant clinical advantage of cryoablation over heat-based modalities is the ability to monitor the evolution of the iceball in real time or near real time with US, CT, and MRI. The iceball identified during monitoring corresponds extremely well with the zone of necrosis observed following the ablation [10,44,45]. Real-time monitoring of the iceball allows adjustments to be made in the duration of the ablation and the intensity of freezing of individual cryoprobes, thus sculpting the iceball to obtain adequate ablation margins while avoiding excessive ablation of normal tissue and/or injury to adjacent structures.

MRI is perhaps the optimal modality for monitoring cryoablation, as the inherent tissue contrast between the tumor and normal hepatic parenchyma allows better differentiation of the tumor margin than non-contrast CT or US. Also, the iceball demonstrates a prominent signal void during freezing, which allows relatively precise matching of the ablation zone to the tumor margin [44]. CT and US also demonstrate excellent agreement between the position of the iceball seen on imaging and the subsequent zone of necrosis [10,45]. On CT, the iceball is identified as a low-attenuation focus, near water density, making it very conspicuous compared to the adjacent normal liver parenchyma. In contrast, differentiation of the tumor from normal parenchyma can be difficult on non-contrast CT, complicating the monitoring of the ablation if CT guidance is utilized. US has several advantages when utilized for targeting and monitoring of cryoablation. During targeting, US allows continuous monitoring of the position of the probe. During the ablation process, the iceball produces a hyperechoic line along its anterior margin and near-complete reflection of the ultrasound beam. This results in obscuration of the margin of the iceball opposite the transducer. Although multiple sonographic windows can be used to evaluate the iceball, it can be difficult to confirm the posterior margin of the ablation (Fig. 10.3). Therefore, in our practice, probe placement is typically completed under ultrasound guidance, while the evolution of the ablation is monitored with intermittent CT.

Real-time monitoring of the iceball allows the use of one of the unique benefits of cryoablation. The size and shape of the iceball can be controlled both through the placement of the individual cryoprobes and by adjusting the relative power and active cooling time of each probe. This allows a degree of precision that is not possible with the heat-based ablation modalities (Fig. 10.4). This precision can also be exploited to protect adjacent structures. In cases where manipulating the iceball shape is not necessary, the 100% power output should be used, since rapid freezing results in the formation of intracellular ice and the subsequent disruption of membranes, which is more highly cytotoxic. Rapid rates of temperature change have been associated with an increased percentage of cellular death when compared to slower rates of freezing [46].

In addition to adjusting the time, power, and position of cryoprobes, it is typical to perform multiple freeze cycles. A double freeze–thaw cycle results in a

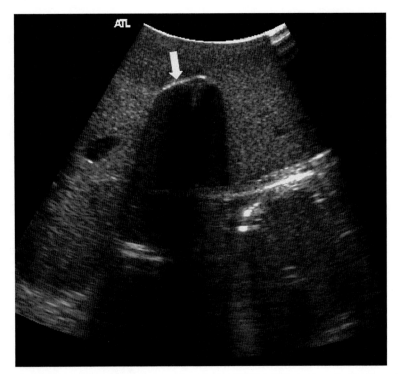

Figure 10.3 Intraoperative ultrasound image during iceball formation. The leading edge of the iceball is identified as a hyperechoic line (arrow) and there is dense posterior shadowing. As a result, the more distal aspects of the cryoablation zone can be difficult to assess.

faster rate of freezing on subsequent freezes and a larger zone of necrosis than a single freeze of similar total duration [47]. A 10-minute freeze, 5-minute thaw, and repeat 10-minute freeze is a common protocol. Longer durations of freezing and more than two freeze–thaw cycles result in increased ablation margin, but with exponentially smaller gains with each freeze [48]. Therefore, if a portion of the tumor is untreated after two freeze–thaw cycles, it is generally preferable to place another cryoprobe into the untreated area rather than increase the number or duration of freeze cycles. Note that frozen tissue will deflect additional cryoprobes, and the iceball may need to be thawed before additional probes can be placed.

At our institution, if there is no contraindication, a contrast-enhanced CT is performed at the end of the ablation. The goal of this CT is to identify residual disease or complications. This allows for immediate revision of the ablation

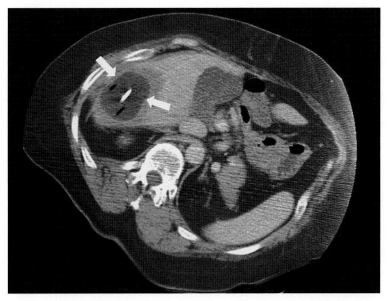

Figure 10.4 Non-contrast CT image through the abdomen during cryoablation. The iceball is well seen as a low-attenuation (HU approximate 0) area on CT imaging. This allows precise control of the ablation as the iceball can be monitored and manipulated based upon its size and growth.

margin, or intervention for complications, if necessary. This CT also serves as a valuable reference exam for subsequent follow-up studies.

Periprocedural sedation and pain control

Radiofrequency ablation is often associated with severe pain, making conscious sedation during these procedures challenging. However, cryoablation is associated with relatively little pain and can usually be performed under conscious sedation [49]. Thus patients who may not be candidates for general anesthesia can be considered for cryoablation. Of course, the attendant risks of conscious sedation should also be considered during patient selection. Image-guided ablation in general often requires the patient to be in an awkward position for prolonged periods of time. Therefore, although conscious sedation is generally adequate for cryoablation, general anesthesia should be considered since it can allow a greater degree of comfort. General anesthesia also has the advantage of allowing more reproducible and longer breath-holds, which decreases the risk of patient movement during probe placement. Reproducible breath-holds can be especially important if probe placement is being performed with CT or MRI guidance.

Post-procedure patient management

Post-ablation monitoring and care differ between providers. The majority of the pain associated with cryoablation is often due to body-wall musculoskeletal pain related to the awkward positions required and the percutaneous punctures, rather than to the ablation itself. Thus renal cryoablation can be performed as an out-patient procedure. However, at our institution, we typically require an overnight inpatient stay following cryoablation, primarily for observation and early identification of any delayed complications. Post-ablation care should include close monitoring for the first 4–6 hours following the procedure, and anti-emetics and intravenous fluids until the patient can tolerate oral intake. Patient-controlled analgesia is generally not required for cryoablation, but can be provided as needed. If an intercostal approach was used, a post-procedure chest radiograph can be performed to evaluate for pneumothorax, but it is not required unless the patient has respiratory symptoms.

Post-procedure alterations in liver aminotransferase levels and platelet counts are common, and should be expected following cryoablation. The degree of the elevation in serum AST has been shown to correlate with the size of the ablation, and a greater increase is seen with double freeze–thaw cycles [50]. A decrease in the platelet count is also encountered in almost all patients (nadir occurs on the third post-ablation day), the severity of which is proportional to the elevation in the AST [51].

Complications

The risks of cryoablation can be divided into those that are inherent to any percutaneous ablation modality, and those that are linked specifically to cryoablation. The rate of procedure-related mortality is low, with one pooled review documenting a 1.6% mortality rate in 869 patients from different series [52]. The most common cause of periprocedural mortality in this review was acute myocardial infarction.

Hemorrhage

Post-procedure hemorrhage is a possibility with any percutaneous liver procedure. In patients with cirrhosis and associated poor hepatic function, the relative decrease in clotting factors can significantly increase the risk of hemorrhage. As a result, the ablation of HCC in the setting of cirrhosis does have an increased, but small, risk of associated hemorrhage. Cryoablation has traditionally been considered to have a higher risk of hemorrhage than the heat-based ablation modalities, due to the inherent cautery associated with heat-based ablations and the lack of cautery associated with cryoablation. However, experimental evaluation in a porcine model failed to demonstrate a significant difference in the hemorrhage associated with a cryoablation performed with a single cryoprobe as compared to RFA performed with a single radiofrequency electrode [53]. Clinically, the risk of major hemorrhage has been shown to be less than 5% in several large series [52,54]. In the most serious cases, hemorrhage occurs in the setting of "cracking" of the liver capsule. Since this is often associated with disruption of the liver capsule, there can be rapid and massive blood loss. Liver "cracking" is rare, and may be related to the mechanical stress imposed by the rapid freeze–thaw cycle. The air–capsule interface present during open procedures may potentiate this effect, although this occurred during percutaneous cryoablation as well [18]. Cracking is most likely to occur during the thawing phase of the treatment. In most cases, post-ablation hemorrhage can be treated with blood transfusions and factor replacement. Rarely, surgical intervention may be required.

Abscess

Cryoablation creates a zone of necrosis within the liver, which can be susceptible to infection. However, the rate of abscess formation is low, and most patients who go on to develop an abscess have easily identifiable risk factors. Patients with a history of a biliary procedure that violates the sphincter of Oddi, such as biliary stent placement, sphincterotomy, or biliary enteric anastamosis or fistulas, are at increased risk of abscess formation following ablation [55]. This is presumably due to colonization of the biliary system by bacteria and retrograde infection of the zone of necrosis. In our experience, patients with biliary–enteric communications are at very high risk of abscess formation, and this can occur following both RFA and cryoablation. These patients usually require placement of long-term drainage catheters into the abscess cavity. Any patient considered for ablation with one of these conditions should be informed that there is a very high likelihood that an abscess will develop and require a drainage catheter.

Less commonly, bacteremia of any cause can seed the ablation site, leading to abscess formation. As a result, it is currently standard practice at our institution to provide patients with a single dose of a first-generation cephalosporin (or alternative antibiotic if allergic) immediately prior to the ablation. If a patient without biliary–enteric communication develops a post-procedure abscess, it can usually be managed with percutaneous aspiration and antibiotic therapy [56].

Tumor lysis syndrome (cryoshock)

Cryoshock is a potentially severe tumor lysis syndrome that is essentially unique to cryoablation. Because cryoablation does not cause cauterization of the vessels in the ablation zone, the necrotic contents of the ablation zone are released into the systemic circulation following thawing and reperfusion at the completion of the ablation. The resulting systemic inflammatory response can be severe, and has been termed "cryoshock." The resulting inflammatory cascade can result in severe coagulopathy, thrombocytopenia, disseminated intravascular coagulation, shock, and multi-organ system failure. Cryoshock is an uncommon complication, occurring in approximately 1% of patients [57]. The risk appears to be related to the volume of liver tissue destroyed. In our experience, patients with HCC in the setting of cirrhosis are at increased risk for cryoshock and liver failure after cryoablation compared to RFA.

Tumor seeding

Tumor seeding is a potential concern with any percutaneous intervention on malignant lesions, including biopsy, RFA and cryoablation. However, the risk is small, approximately 0.5% for RFA in several large case series [58,59] and lower than the risk of tumor seeding during open resection [60,61]. Subcapsular or peripheral lesions with little overlying normal parenchyma are at greater risk of tumor seeding. If possible, the cryoprobe tract should traverse normal parenchyma prior to entering the target lesion. The risk is also thought to be higher with larger probes and multiple punctures.

Post-ablation syndrome

Post-ablation syndrome is a well-described spectrum of symptoms that occur after an ablation. Symptom onset is generally delayed, with onset approximately 3 days after the ablation, and the symptoms generally last up to 5 days. The symptoms include an array of flu-like symptoms such as fever, malaise, chills, nausea, and delayed pain [62]. Although the exact underlying mechanism is unknown, the post-ablation syndrome likely represents a relatively minor manifestation of the systemic inflammatory response seen with cryoshock. These symptoms should not be worrisome for a developing infection or other underlying process unless the patient has other risk factors, associated symptoms, or the fever persists beyond 10 days.

Biliary complications

Biliary complications can be conceptually divided into those involving the peripheral ducts and those involving the central ducts. When small, peripheral bile ducts are involved in the ablation zone, particularly in cases involving ablation of a resection margin, the primary risk is the development of a biloma or biliary fistula. Bilomas occur in approximately 3% of cryoablation cases [52]. Most bilomas and fistulas involving peripheral bile ducts are likely to be clinically silent. Ablation in the central liver carries a risk of stricture or obstruction of the central biliary system, which can be particularly problematic in patients with limited hepatic reserve. Some investigators have suggested that cryoablation is less injurious to the biliary system than heat-based ablation modalities [63,64]. However, one should still be cognizant of the central ducts, and they should not be included in the ablation zone. If this is not possible with RFA or cryoablation, ethanol ablation may be a viable alternative. Ethanol ablation carries a lower risk of biliary injury, but is associated with a greater risk of local recurrence when compared to RFA and generally requires serial injections [65,66].

Follow-up

As discussed previously, imaging follow-up begins immediately following ablation at our institution (assuming no contraindications to IV contrast). At that time, a contrast-enhanced CT is performed to identify any residual tumor and to evaluate for adequate margins. A 1 cm "surgical" margin should be the goal with the ablation of metastatic disease, while a margin somewhat less than 1 cm may be adequate for HCC [36]. This initial CT also serves as a baseline examination for comparison purposes.

It is important to be aware of the appearance of recurrent disease as well as the expected evolution of the ablation zone, since there can be overlap in the imaging manifestations of the two processes. Immediately after the iceball is thawed, contrast-enhanced studies generally demonstrate that the ablation site becomes

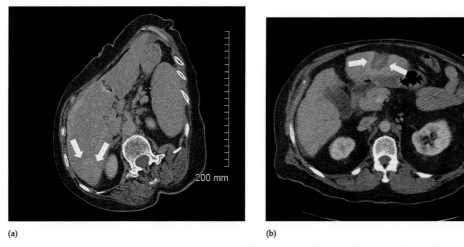

(a)   (b)

Figure 10.5 (a) Contrast-enhanced CT image following cryoablation of hepatic colorectal metastasis. The ablation zone in this patient is higher in attenuation than the adjacent liver. This appearance is sometimes seen following cryoablation and is likely related to reperfusion of the ablation zone following iceball thawing with either contrast enhancement or focal hemorrhage. (b) Contrast-enhanced image through the liver following radio frequency ablation (RFA) of a left-lobe hepatocellular carcinoma. The appearance of the ablation zone after RFA is more predictable, with the area being devascularized and low in attenuation.

hypervascular as the blood flow returns (Fig. 10.5). This is in stark contrast to RFA, where the ablation zone is hypovascular. As a result, enhancement in the cryoablation zone immediately after thawing is not necessarily indicative of residual disease. Over the next several days the vessels in the zone of ablation thrombose and the ablation zone becomes hypovascular, often with a surrounding confluent and uniform hypervascular rim during the acute inflammatory phase. This hypervascular rim should not be confused with the nodular, irregular pattern of hypervascular enhancement seen with residual HCC (Fig. 10.6). If nodular areas of hypervascular enhancement are identified, this should be presumed to represent residual or recurrent disease in cases of HCC. This should be differentiated from the well-marginated, geographic zones of enhancement that can be seen along the border of the ablation zone, thought to arise from small-vessel changes and vascular shunt formation following the ablation [67,68]. A careful search for metachronous disease is also important, as 50% of patients who have undergone resection for HCC will develop a second site of disease within 3 years [54,69].

Identification of recurrent or residual metastatic disease is more difficult, as the initial tumor is often hypovascular with an appearance very similar to the ablation

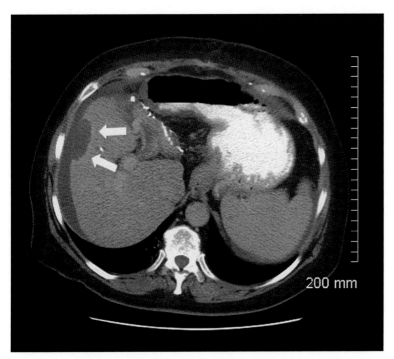

Figure 10.6 Contrast-enhanced CT image through the abdomen 1 month after cryoablation of a right-lobe colorectal metastasis. Along the periphery of the cryoablation site in the right lobe of the liver there is a thin smooth rim of hypervascular enhancement (arrows). This is a normal post-ablation finding and should not be considered evidence for recurrence. A more nodular pattern of enhancement is more concerning and could indicate tumor recurrence.

zone on contrast-enhanced CT. In cases of metastatic disease, landmarks and subtle attenuation differences are often the only imaging manifestation of residual or recurrent disease. Multiple studies have shown that the natural evolution of the ablation zone is a slow decrease in size in the months and years following ablation [70]. Therefore, if the ablation zone remains stable or increases in size, or if there are asymmetric changes in appearance, this should be considered highly suspicious for recurrent disease.

Conclusion

Image-guided tumor ablation is a rapidly evolving minimally invasive technique that is becoming increasingly utilized and accepted for the treatment of various oncologic and benign processes. Tumor ablation can be accomplished with multiple different modalities, including heat-based ablation modalities, chemical ablative techniques, and cryoablation. The different techniques have their own unique advantages and disadvantages, which a physician needs to be aware of prior to performing these procedures. Patient-care decisions in our center regarding the use of surgery, cryotherapy, radiofrequency ablation, and/or intra-arterial therapies are made using a consensus approach with the involved clinical services. Each case is discussed with the clinician and usually presented in a multidisciplinary conference setting, and the decision as to which therapy to utilize is based on the tumor size and location, histology, and associated comorbidities. Since there are no definitive comparative trials between the different locoregional therapies, decisions are also made with deference to physician experience and preference. In general, patients with lesions > 5 cm in diameter, lesions in a location that requires a more precise ablation, lesions adjacent to large vessels (> 3–4 mm) that might represent a significant "heat sink," and lesions ablated in the operating room are treated with cryoablation. We do not utilize cryoablation in cirrhotic patients with hepatocellular carcinoma due to the presumed increased risk of hemorrhage and liver "cracking." All other lesions targeted for local therapy are considered for either radiofrequency ablation or cryoablation. Unfortunately, there are few comparative data to determine the survival and recurrence rates of cryoablation patients in comparison with other locoregional treatment modalities. Additionally, most cryoablation studies are performed in a highly selected patient population and are associated with a significant selection bias. This is a problem with most ablation literature to this point. Local recurrence occurs in a minority of cases and is highly dependent on the tumor type, size, and location, but patients with HCC in the setting of cirrhosis, and metastatic lesions from distant primaries, often have metachronous lesions, which may ultimately limit long-term survival. In this chapter we have reviewed the indications, techniques, and management of patients undergoing image-guided cryoablation of liver masses.

REFERENCES

1. El-Serag HB, Mason AC. Rising incidence of hepatocellular carcinoma in the United States. *N Engl J Med* 1999; **340**: 745–50.
2. Davila JA, Morgan RO, Shaib Y, McGlynn KA, El-Serag HB. Hepatitis C infection and the increasing incidence of hepatocellular carcinoma: a population-based study. *Gastroenterology* 2004; **127**: 1372–80.

3. Winter TC, Laeseke PF, Lee FT Jr. Focal tumor ablation: a new era in cancer therapy. *Ultrasound Q* 2006; **22**: 195–217.

4. Cagol PP, Pasqual E, Bacchetti S. Natural history of the neoplastic locoregional disease: clinical and pathological patterns. *J Exp Clin Cancer Res* 2003; **22** (4 Suppl): 1–4.

5. Ries LA, Krapcho M, Mariotto A, *et al.*, eds. *SEER Cancer Statistics Review, 1975–2004*. Bethesda, MD: National Cancer Institute, 2007.

6. Scheele J, Stang R, Altendorf-Hofmann A, Paul M. Resection of colorectal liver metastases. *World J Surg* 1995; **19**: 59–71.

7. Hoffmann NE, Bischof JC. The cryobiology of cryosurgical injury. *Urology* 2002; **60** (Suppl 1): 40–9.

8. Zacarian SA. The observation of freeze–thaw cycles upon cancer-cell suspensions. *J Dermatol Surg Oncol* 1977; **3**: 173–4.

9. Rubinsky B, Lee CY, Bastacky J, Onik G. The process of freezing and the mechanism of damage during hepatic cryosurgery. *Cryobiology* 1990; **27**: 85–97.

10. Weber SM, Lee FT Jr, Warner TF, Chosy SG, Mahvi DM. Hepatic cryoablation: US monitoring of extent of necrosis in normal pig liver. *Radiology* 1998; **207**: 73–7.

11. Zhang BH, Yang BH, Tang ZY. Randomized controlled trial of screening for hepatocellular carcinoma. *J Cancer Res Clin Oncol* 2004; **130**: 417–22.

12. Colli A, Fraquelli M, Casazza G, *et al.* Accuracy of ultrasonography, spiral CT, magnetic resonance, and alpha-fetoprotein in diagnosing hepatocellular carcinoma: a systematic review. *Am J Gastroenterol* 2006; **101**: 513–23.

13. Duffy JP, Vardanian A, Benjamin E, *et al.* Liver transplantation criteria for hepatocellular carcinoma should be expanded: a 22-year experience with 467 patients at UCLA. *Ann Surg* 2007; **246**: 502–11.

14. Baccarani U, Benzoni E, Adani GL, *et al.* Superiority of transplantation versus resection for the treatment of small hepatocellular carcinoma. *Transplant Proc* 2007; **39**: 1898–900.

15. Lai EC, Fan ST, Lo CM, *et al.* Hepatic resection for hepatocellular carcinoma: an audit of 343 patients. *Ann Surg* 1995; **221**: 291–8.

16. Llovet J, Ricci S, Mazzaferro V, *et al.* for the SHARP Investigators Study Group. Sorafenib improves survival in advanced hepatocellular carcinoma (HCC): results of a phase III randomized placebo-controlled trial (SHARP trial). *J Clin Oncol* 2007; **25** (18S): LBA1 (2007 ASCO Annual Meeting Proceedings Part I).

17. Adam R, Akpinar E, Johann M, *et al.* Place of cryosurgery in the treatment of malignant liver tumors. *Ann Surg* 1997; **225**: 39–50.

18. Xu KC, Niu LZ, He WB, *et al.* Percutaneous cryoablation in combination with ethanol injection for unresectable hepatocellular carcinoma. *World J Gastroenterol* 2003; **9**: 2686–9.

19. Tait IS, Yong SM, Cuschieri SA. Laparoscopic in situ ablation of liver cancer with cryotherapy and radiofrequency ablation. *Br J Surg* 2002; **89**: 1613–19.

20. Gouillat C, Manganas D, Saguier G, Duque-Campos R, Berard P. Resection of hepatocellular carcinoma in cirrhotic patients: longterm results of a prospective study. *J Am Coll Surg* 1999; **189**: 282–90.

21. Lau WY, Leung TW, Yu SC, Ho SK. Percutaneous local ablative therapy for hepatocellular carcinoma: a review and look into the future. *Ann Surg* 2003; **237**: 171–9.

22. Lawes D, Chopada A, Gillams A, Lees W, Taylor I. Radiofrequency ablation (RFA) as a cytoreductive strategy for hepatic metastasis from breast cancer. *Ann R Coll Surg Engl* 2006; **88**: 639–42.

23. Livraghi T, Goldberg SN, Solbiati L, *et al.* Percutaneous radio-frequency ablation of liver metastases from breast cancer: initial experience in 24 patients. *Radiology* 2001; **220**: 145–9.

24. Alseidi A, Helton WS, Espat NJ. Does the literature support an indication for hepatic metastasectomy other than for colorectal primary? *J Gastrointest Surg* 2006; **10**: 99–104.

25. Ahmad A, Chen SL, Bilchik AJ. Role of repeated hepatectomy in the multimodal treatment of hepatic colorectal metastases. *Arch Surg* 2007; **142**: 526–32.

26. Ravikumar TS, Kane R, Cady B, *et al.* A 5-year study of cryosurgery in the treatment of liver tumors. *Arch Surg* 1991; **126**: 1520–4.

27. Tuttle TM, Curley SA, Roh MS. Repeat hepatic resection as effective treatment of recurrent colorectal liver metastases. *Ann Surg Oncol* 1997; **4**: 125–30.

28. Pawlik TM, Choti MA. Surgical therapy for colorectal metastases to the liver. *J Gastrointest Surg* 2007; **11**: 1057–77.

29. Stangl R, Altendorf-Hofmann A, Charnley RM, Scheele J. Factors influencing the natural history of colorectal liver metastases. *Lancet* 1994; **343**: 1405–10.

30. Scheele J, Altendorf-Hofmann A. Resection of colorectal liver metastases. *Langenbecks Arch Surg* 1999; **384**: 313–27.

31. Ballantyne GH, Quin J. Surgical treatment of liver metastases in patients with colorectal cancer. *Cancer* 1993; **71** (12 Suppl): 4252–66.

32. Aggarwal S, Chu E. Current therapies for advanced colorectal cancer. *Oncology* (Williston Park) 2005; **19**: 589–95.

33. Goldberg RM. Advances in the treatment of metastatic colorectal cancer. *Oncologist* 2005; **10** (Suppl 3): 40–8.

34. Emmanouilides C, Sfakiotaki G, Androulakis N, *et al.* Front-line bevacizumab in combination with oxaliplatin, leucovorin and 5-fluorouracil (FOLFOX) in patients with metastatic colorectal cancer: a multicenter phase II study. *BMC Cancer* 2007; **7**: 91.

35. Seifert JK, Morris DL. Indicators of recurrence following cryotherapy for hepatic metastases from colorectal cancer. *Br J Surg* 1999; **86**: 234–40.

36. Livraghi T, Goldberg SN, Lazzaroni S, *et al.* Small hepatocellular carcinoma: treatment with radio-frequency ablation versus ethanol injection. *Radiology* 1999; **210**: 655–61.

37. Wang H, Littrup PJ, Duan Y, *et al.* Thoracic masses treated with percutaneous cryotherapy: initial experience with more than 200 procedures. *Radiology* 2005; **235**: 289–98.

38. Muller-Schweinitzer E. Arterial smooth muscle function after prolonged exposure to a medium containing dimethyl sulfoxide (Me_2SO) and storage at −196 degrees C. *Cryobiology* 1994; **31**: 330–5.

39. Koda M, Ueki M, Maeda Y, *et al.* Percutaneous sonographically guided radiofrequency ablation with artificial pleural effusion for hepatocellular carcinoma located under the diaphragm. *AJR Am J Roentgenol* 2004; **183**: 583–8.

40. Toyoda M, Kakizaki S, Horiuchi K, *et al.* Computed tomography-guided transpulmonary radiofrequency ablation for hepatocellular carcinoma located in hepatic dome. *World J Gastroenterol* 2006; **12**: 608–11.

41. Adam R, Hagopian EJ, Linhares M, *et al.* A comparison of percutaneous cryosurgery and percutaneous radiofrequency for unresectable hepatic malignancies. *Arch Surg* 2002; **137**: 1332–40.

42. Cervone A, Sardi A, Conaway GL. Intraoperative ultrasound (IOUS) is essential in the management of metastatic colorectal liver lesions. *Am Surg* 2000; **66**: 611–15.

43. Leen E, Ceccotti P, Moug SJ, *et al.* Potential value of contrast-enhanced intraoperative ultrasonography during partial hepatectomy for metastases: an essential investigation before resection? *Ann Surg* 2006; **243**: 236–40.

44. Silverman SG, Tuncali K, Adams DF, *et al.* MR imaging-guided percutaneous cryotherapy of liver tumors: initial experience. *Radiology* 2000; **217**: 657–64.

45. Lee FT Jr, Chosy SG, Littrup PJ, *et al.* CT-monitored percutaneous cryoablation in a pig liver model: pilot study. *Radiology* 1999; **211**: 687–92.

46. Neel HB 3rd, Ketcham AS, Hammond WG. Requisites for successful cryogenic surgery of cancer. *Arch Surg* 1971; **102**: 45–8.

47. Mala T, Edwin B, Tillung T, *et al.* Percutaneous cryoablation of colorectal liver metastases: potentiated by two consecutive freeze–thaw cycles. *Cryobiology* 2003; **46**: 99–102.

48. Cooper IS, Hirose T. Application of cryogenic surgery to resection of parenchymal organs. *N Engl J Med* 1966; **274**: 15–18.

49. Allaf ME, Varkarakis IM, Bhayani SB, *et al.* Pain control requirements for percutaneous ablation of renal tumors: cryoablation versus radiofrequency ablation – initial observations. *Radiology* 2005; **237**: 366–70.

50. Stewart GJ, Preketes A, Horton M, *et al.* Hepatic cryotherapy: double-freeze cycles achieve greater hepatocellular injury in man. *Cryobiology* 1995; **32**: 215–19.

51. McKinnon JG, Temple WJ, Wiseman DA, Saliken JC. Cryosurgery for malignant tumours of the liver. *Can J Surg* 1996; **39**: 401–6.

52. Seifert JK, Junginger T, Morris DL. A collective review of the world literature on hepatic cryotherapy. *J R Coll Surg Edinb* 1998; **43**: 141–54.

53. Shock SA, Laeseke PF, Sampson LA, *et al.* Hepatic hemorrhage caused by percutaneous tumor ablation: radiofrequency ablation versus cryoablation in a porcine model. *Radiology* 2005; **236**: 125–31.

54. Zhou XD, Tang ZY, Yang BH, *et al.* Experience of 1000 patients who underwent hepatectomy for small hepatocellular carcinoma. *Cancer* 2001; **91**: 1479–86.

55. Riley DK, Babinchak TJ, Zemel R, *et al.* Infectious complications of hepatic cryosurgery. *Clin Infect Dis* 1997; **24**: 1001–3.

56. Yu SC, Ho SS, Lau WY, *et al.* Treatment of pyogenic liver abscess: prospective randomized comparison of catheter drainage and needle aspiration. *Hepatology* 2004; **39**: 932–8.

57. Seifert JK, Morris DL. World survey on the complications of hepatic and prostate cryotherapy. *World J Surg* 1999; **23**: 109–14.

58. Livraghi T, Solbiati L, Meloni MF, *et al.* Treatment of focal liver tumors with percutaneous radio-frequency ablation: complications encountered in a multicenter study. *Radiology* 2003; **226**: 441–51.

59. de Baere T, Risse O, Kuoch V, *et al.* Adverse events during radiofrequency treatment of 582 hepatic tumors. *AJR Am J Roentgenol* 2003; **181**: 695–700.

60. Yeh CN, Chen MF, Jeng LB. Resection of peritoneal implantation from hepatocellular carcinoma. *Ann Surg Oncol* 2002; **9**: 863–8.

61. Cha C, Fong Y, Jarnagin WR, *et al.* Predictors and patterns of recurrence after resection of hepatocellular carcinoma. *J Am Coll Surg* 2003; **197**: 753–8.

62. Dodd GD 3rd, Napier D, Schoolfield JD, Hubbard L. Percutaneous radiofrequency ablation of hepatic tumors: postablation syndrome. *AJR Am J Roentgenol* 2005; **185**: 51–7.

63. Kahlenberg MS, Volpe C, Klippenstein DL, *et al.* Clinicopathologic effects of cryotherapy on hepatic vessels and bile ducts in a porcine model. *Ann Surg Oncol* 1998; **5**: 713–18.

64. Akahane M, Koga H, Kato N, *et al.* Complications of percutaneous radiofrequency ablation for hepato-cellular carcinoma: imaging spectrum and management. *Radiographics* 2005; **25** (Suppl 1): S57–68.

65. Lencioni R, Cioni D, Crocetti L, *et al.* Early-stage hepatocellular carcinoma in patients with cirrhosis: long-term results of percutaneous image-guided radiofrequency ablation. *Radiology* 2005; **234**: 961–7.

66. Lin SM, Lin CJ, Lin CC, *et al.* Randomised controlled trial comparing percutaneous radio-frequency thermal ablation, percutaneous ethanol injection, and percutaneous acetic acid injection to treat hepatocellular carcinoma of 3 cm or less. *Gut* 2005; **54**: 1151–6.

67. Kuszyk BS, Choti MA, Urban BA, *et al.* Hepatic tumors treated by cryosurgery: normal CT appearance. *AJR Am J Roentgenol* 1996; **166**: 363–8.

68. McLoughlin RF, Saliken JF, McKinnon G, *et al.* CT of the liver after cryotherapy of hepatic metastases: imaging findings. *AJR Am J Roentgenol* 1995; **165**: 329–32.

69. Sugimachi K, Maehara S, Tanaka S, *et al.* Repeat hepatectomy is the most useful treatment for recurrent hepatocellular carcinoma. *J Hepatobiliary Pancreat Surg* 2001; **8**: 410–16.

70. Dromain C, de Baere T, Elias D, *et al.* Hepatic tumors treated with percutaneous radio-frequency ablation: CT and MR imaging follow-up. *Radiology* 2002; **223**: 255–62.

11

Considerations in setting up a radiofrequency ablation service: how we do it

Fadi M. El-Merhi, Gerald D. Dodd, and Linda G. Hubbard

Introduction

Interventional oncology (IO) has emerged as a major subspecialty in the medical and surgical treatment of patients with cancer. As a discipline it encompasses the diagnosis, treatment, and follow-up of patients with a wide range of cancers involving but not limited to the liver, kidneys, prostate, lungs, and breast. Specific procedures include biopsy, thermal and chemical ablation, transcatheter techniques such as chemoembolization and radioembolization, and high-intensity focused ultrasound. At the highest level of practice it involves a team of subspecialists who can provide the full spectrum of treatment options; at a minimum it requires a medical practitioner who is skilled in at least one of the treatment techniques and is dedicated to the evaluation, treatment, and follow-up of patients. Interventional oncology should not be practiced as a single-encounter event, wherein the only role of the IO physician is the performance of an interventional procedure; it is a discipline that requires the practitioner to become an actively engaged member of the patient's healthcare team. Over the last 10–15 years there have been many changes and improvements in the treatment of patients with all types of cancer. Chemotherapy, surgery, and radiation therapy have made significant strides in the treatment of disease that, in the past, was thought to be untreatable. In this chapter we will specifically discuss how to set up a radiofrequency ablation (RFA) service, and how to integrate it with the multidisciplinary practice of cancer treatment. However, many of the points of discussion are equally applicable to the creation of a global IO practice. For example, several years ago, if a patient presented with three or four liver metastases from colon cancer, he or she may have been offered only one line of chemotherapy, without much real improvement in survival. The radiologist's role, if any, was to read the CT scan, which probably would have been dictated as

Interventional Radiological Treatment of Liver Tumors, ed. Andy Adam and Peter R. Mueller.
Published by Cambridge University Press. © Cambridge University Press 2009.

"the liver contains multiple metastases." Now it is imperative for the radiologist to be specific in the number and location of the metastases. The patient may have chemotherapy, but it will be a multi-drug regimen. In addition, the number and location of the metastases and their size will determine whether the patient undergoes surgery alone, surgery combined with RFA, or even chemoembolization. The radiologist needs to have a much more active role in the diagnosis and treatment of these and other types of tumors.

Training for the radiologist in ablation

Operating an RFA service requires a unique skill set. It includes being an excellent diagnostic radiologist; a skilled proceduralist with good hand–eye coordination; a good clinician who is comfortable managing patients and post-therapeutic complications; and a good communicator who enjoys working with patients, support staff, and referring physicians. Ideally, practitioners performing RFA should be fellowship-trained in IO and capable of running a full-spectrum IO practice. For those interventional radiologists who graduated before IO became established, a visiting professorship or mini-fellowship in RFA should be taken before attempting to start an RFA practice.

A practitioner who wishes to start an RFA service must be fully versed in the spectrum of therapeutic options available to treat a given tumor, as well as the indication and contraindications of each treatment option. A thorough knowledge of the anesthetic options, image-guidance techniques, RFA equipment options and performance parameters, RFA treatment strategies, complications of RFA, and post-RFA management protocols is essential. Specific procedural skills that must be mastered before performing RFA include the ability to use image guidance to position RFA probes accurately within tumors, the ability to reposition RFA probes within specified portions of large tumors to execute composite ablations necessary to treat large tumors, and the ability to use the RFA probe to cauterize the probe track to prevent bleeding and minimize tumor seeding.

The modalities used to guide placement of the RFA probes varies with the disease treated. Many radiologists use ultrasound for small, peripheral liver lesions (primary or secondary tumors) and CT for treatments in difficult-to-see liver lesions, kidneys, lungs, and bone. Because ablation covers many organ system areas, several different approaches have been instituted in the United States. In some departments, based on separating cross-sectional interventional procedures from vascular (fluoroscopic) procedures, an abdominal or chest radiologist might perform treatments in the liver, kidney, bone, etc. However, in a department in which all the intervention is incorporated in the vascular-intervention division, the interventionalist performs all of the ablations. What is clear is that individuals who perform these procedures must be facile in image-guided procedures and cross-sectional imaging. Because the pre-procedure imaging and post-procedure imaging can be difficult, these cases must always be read by individuals who have an understanding of how RFA can affect the organ treated. This understanding will prevent misreadings.

In addition, as the field of ablation has evolved, there has been considerable research on combination therapies such as chemoembolization, and individuals who perform ablation need to understand their role. It is not reasonable to expect that one individual can be an expert in all of these areas without exposure through fellowships, courses, and seminars, as the field is changing rapidly. Clearly, an interventional background is essential, as patient care is a *sine qua non* of this specialty.

Hospital admitting privileges

In many practices in the United States, the interventionalist has admitting privileges. Many interventional socities encourage this approach. While most of the procedures can be performed on an outpatient basis, there will be patients who require overnight observation or have a complication that will require extended admission to the hospital. It is imperative, if you do not have admitting privileges, that you establish relationships with your referrals to admit a patient. In many cases admitting a patient with renal failure, and who has had a renal RFA, to a kidney specialist is better for the patient than admitting to a radiologist. Certainly, these are relationships that need to be worked out prior to starting a service. Also, the radiologist needs to be actively involved with the patient's care, even if he or she is not the primary admitter. Some would argue that radiologists lose their "stature" with their fellow physicians if they don't take "full care" of a patient with complications. This is not necessarily true, as the interaction of all physicians revolves around mutual respect. This applies to all interventional procedures, and to have a referring physician help you with patient care, as long as this is worked out prior to starting a procedure, may be best for the patient.

Setting up a clinic

Having a dedicated office or sharing one with another clinical subspecialty is an essential element of an RFA practice. An office should include a waiting area and an examination room. The arrangement of the office space should be set up to maintain patient privacy and confidentiality. The examination room should be equipped to allow the performance of an appropriate medical history and physical examination. View-boxes and a monitor should be present so that a patient's imaging studies can be reviewed. Ideally, both should be positioned so that the imaging studies can be reviewed with the patient. The room should be large enough to accommodate the attendance of at least one other family member. The RFA procedural room can be within the office structure as long as there is an accessible recovery room, as both go hand in hand; otherwise, the procedural room may be in a hospital or surgery center.

A clinic is helpful for pre- and post-visits. As RFA procedures lead to "longitudinal care" for patients, having a central area to assist coordinate care is essential. An office requires considerable support, both by the administration of your department or hospital, and by individuals who are hired to work in it.

Professional team

The most important resource of any clinical practice is its professional team. This includes receptionists, nurses, anesthesiologists, imaging technologists, and consultant physicians. All must be dedicated to providing the highest-quality patient care and timely service, for it is the experience of the patient and referring physician that ultimately determines the success of the practice. On a day-to-day basis, having an experienced nurse coordinator or physician assistant working hand in hand with the interventional radiologist is crucial to the process. There is a great deal of coordination required with RFA patients. For example, if the patient is on anticoagulants, has an artificial pacemaker, or needs anesthesia, a number of issues must be resolved. If radiologists attempt to do this by themselves, they will be bogged down in administrative issues and will not have the time to build the practice. Scheduling, pre-authorization of forms for insurance companies, and other insurance issues can be coordinated by the "office team." They can also participate with the interventional radiologist in forming a clinical assessment and plan, order follow-up laboratory tests or imaging studies, schedule the procedure date, refer the patient for pre-treatment assessment by an anesthesiologist, schedule follow-up appointments, and manage a patient's chart. An anesthesia team that will be helping the interventional radiologist during the procedure, and a recovery nurse who will take care of the patient during the post-procedure phase, are all part of the professional team. Lastly, it is important to develop a list of colleagues on whom you can call for consultation regarding the management of patients with acute medical conditions. These may include surgeons, in the event of a surgical emergency, or medical subspecialists such as hospitalists, gastroenterologists, or nephrologists. Many of these physicians will already be in the system as referrers, but it is helpful to keep them up to date about the patient's course after the procedure, follow-up imaging, etc. It is clear from studies from a number of centers that a complete well-functioning RFA service cannot be obtained without consideration of a clinic and supporting staff.

Billing team

Professional billing for these procedures obviously varies, not only by the country where the procedure is performed (e.g., United Kingdom vs. United States) but also by where in the country it is performed, particularly in the United States (e.g., Northeast vs. West). In many instances the billing system and bureaucracy is arcane and difficult to unravel.

However, it is important to have a dedicated billing team that can manage the complexity of the billing process. These individuals are essential to the financial success of the operation and should not be left to work in a vacuum. IO physicians should work closely with the billing team to assure that all aspects of a patient's care are correctly documented and billed. Most patient encounters will generate evaluation and management codes (in the United States for physical exams), as well as imaging and laboratory codes [2]. These codes are separate from the ones that describe the interventional procedure, and they are important in identifying physician status (treating vs. consultant), patient status (inpatient vs. outpatient), encounter time, and service complexity [3]. Often the companies selling the probes have some individual (in the United States) who can help also with sorting out the billing issues.

Certainly, making money on these procedures is important. But, the interventionalist must realize the value of having such a service, the considerable addition of imaging studies pre- and post-procedure, and the marketing aspect of having someone who can treat these patients with significant tumors.

Marketing and building referrals

Marketing is crucial to the development of an RFA practice. Marketing can refer to both "internal" and "external" marketing. For external publicity, referring doctors and the public must be informed about the services being provided. In this age of globalization, a website is essential. The site should describe the RFA procedure, eligibility criteria, and how to initiate a referral or consultation. A brief description of each member of the professional team and their respective roles helps to personalize the page. Animated movie clips are very useful for demonstrating the key elements of the RFA procedure. Other conventional methods of building a practice include mailing notification letters and brochures to potential future referring physicians, medical directors, and practice managers in the same city or geographic region. More aggressive techniques for building a practice include placing advertisements in the local newspapers, county and state medical society newsletters or magazines, and on regional billboards. Promotional spots can be purchased on local radio stations [4].

Internal marketing to physicians within the hospital sphere is probably a better way to start. Interventional oncology physicians, who are also practicing diagnostic radiologists or who are part of a diagnostic radiology group, can use the primary interpretation process as a very effective method by which to build an RFA practice. As appropriate, patients for RFA are identified during the routine interpretation of diagnostic imaging studies; either a call can be placed to the referring physician to discuss the patient's potential treatment, or a statement regarding the appropriateness and availability of RFA can be added to the diagnostic report. In a hospital setting, IO physicians should give presentations on RFA at grand rounds of the different clinical services that manage patients with cancer, such as hepatology, medical oncology, surgical oncology, pulmonology, urology, and primary care. They should participate regularly in the multi-specialty tumor board, as it is there that the plan for the treatment of a patient is often decided. If the IO physician is present at the tumor board meeting, and can actively discuss the pros and cons of the various treatment options with his colleagues, his recognition as a valuable colleague will be greatly enhanced and his ability to direct appropriate referrals to his service will increase significantly. This type of internal marketing can be quite effective, but is both time-consuming and may take the practicing IO radiologist away from other duties, such as reading CTs, fluoroscopy, etc. A commitment of the practice or radiologic group is essential for this type of practice to work, as it may take a considerable amount of time to initiate.

Communication

Once the referral pathway is created, it is essential that the physician–patient and physician–physician relationships be carefully managed through both the pre- and post-procedural phases of medical care [5]. Communication with both patients and referring physicians is the foundation for building and maintaining a strong referral pattern. All encounters with a patient should be documented and followed up by timely personal letters to the referring physician and possibly the patient. Patients should be afforded sufficient time in clinic to fully discuss their condition, treatment options, potential complications, and expected outcome. They should be actively involved in the decisions made regarding their medical care. If a patient is admitted to the hospital, daily rounds should be made by the IO physician, even if the patient is admitted to a different service. Biopsy results and interpretations of imaging studies should be sent directly to the referring physician and discussed with the patient. All imaging studies performed after RFA treatment should be reviewed by the IO physician, including those performed at outside institutions, with reports sent to the referring physician. A full-time nurse coordinator is essential to establishing a strong line of communication with referring physicians and patients.

The most difficult aspect of this process is that it requires a different type of radiologic practice than usually performed. If the radiologist performing the RFA does not incorporate a full-time commitment to pre- and postoperative care, follow-up, rounds, and the associated ancillary personnel to accomplish this, the program will not succeed.

Patient management

Typically the first encounter with a potential RFA patient starts without the patient present, as a review of the patient's most recent imaging studies and pertinent clinical history. This consultation can be initiated by a referring physician or directly by a patient. A nurse practitioner or physician assistant is an ideal person to field these consults and to organize the data and images for review with the IO physician. During the review, the patient's data are evaluated to determine if he or she is a potential candidate for RFA. The result of this review should be reported to the referring physician or directly to the patient if self-referred. In academic centers this process may lead to a review of the patient at a multidisciplinary tumor board. Patients who are deemed to be viable candidates for RFA should be scheduled for their first clinic visit.

The initial meeting with the patient should take place in the IO physician's office. The nurse practitioner, physician assistant, or IO physician should take a complete medical history and perform a physical examination. The IO physician should discuss the appropriateness of RFA as a treatment option with the patient, as well as the risks, benefits, outcomes, and possible alternatives to RFA. If the IO physician is planning to use ultrasound as the imaging-guidance technique for the RFA procedure, an ultrasound study should be performed to confirm that the tumor is visible by sonography and that a safe approach exists. All necessary additional imaging or laboratory tests, as well as any needed consultations such as with anesthesiology or cardiology, should be discussed with the patient and scheduled. Medications that need to be discontinued prior to the RFA procedure should be discussed with the patient and possibly with the referring physician. If a different treatment appears more appropriate than RFA, this should be discussed with the patient and the referring physician. If a referral is needed to another specialist it is helpful and greatly appreciated if this action is facilitated by the IO physician or support staff. In all instances the patient's care should be expedited. For patients from out of town it is very helpful to orchestrate their care such that the evaluation process and treatment can be performed in one visit. If a patient appears uncomfortable with the care that an IO physician has recommended, the patient should be offered a referral for a second opinion.

On the day of the RFA procedure, the patient should be instructed to arrive at the hospital several hours before the procedure. This will give the patient enough time to go through admissions and to be seen by the anesthesiology service, if they are going to participate in the procedure. Blood products can be ordered as necessary and the patient can be typed and crossed. The anesthesia team can take care of obtaining IV access, placing the patient on a monitor, and gaining airway control. At the same time, the IO team can start setting up the RFA generator, identifying the ablation probes that may be used, and pulling up the pertinent imaging studies on a nearby accessible PACS or film-panel. After identifying the tumor(s) to be treated by the imaging system that is going to be used to guide the RFA, the procedure can start (specific techniques of the procedure are discussed in Chapter 8). After the procedure is done and no acute complications are identified, the patient should be transferred to a recovery room for observation. It is advisable to meet with the family members immediately after the procedure to discuss the outcome of the procedure and any potential complications that might have occurred during the procedure. The information should be discussed with the patient after recovery from sedation.

Post-procedural follow-up

Keeping your patient and referring physician informed in the post-procedural phase is an important milestone in developing a successful clinical practice. The patient's reports and data should be communicated to the referring physician. At the same time, each new patient should be entered into a clinical tracking program. Immediate follow-up should include daily phone calls for the first week or until the patient is doing well. The patient should return to the IO clinic at 1 week and again at 1 month after the procedure for a post-RFA assessment. Both the serial phone calls and the clinic visit can be performed by the nurse practitioner or the physician assistant. A baseline CT scan or MRI should be performed at some specific time after the procedure, as dictated by individual protocols set up by the IO division. Serial cross-sectional imaging should be performed according to the following schedule or one similar to it: every 3 months for the first year; every 6 months for the second year; and annually thereafter. It is imperative that the IO team remind the patient of his/her scheduled imaging studies, and that the imaging studies be obtained for review by the IO physician. If the follow-up imaging studies show recurrence of tumor, then the patient should be scheduled for a clinic visit to discuss the findings and the treatment options. Once again it is vital that all findings and plans be reported to and/or discussed with the referring physician.

Summary

The structure and operation of an RFA practice following the guidelines that have been described above will send a message to a local medical community that the practice is committed to providing high-quality medical care for patients that meets or exceeds the standards in the medical community. Both patients and referring physicians will recognize the quality and user-friendliness of the practice, with the result being the creation of a strong RFA practice with a broad referral network.

REFERENCES

1. Knaub J. The doctor is in: clinical IR practice means setting up an office. *Radiology Today* 2006; **7** (9): 10.
2. Siskin GP, Bagla S, Sansivero GE, Mitchell NL. The interventional radiology clinic: key ingredients for success. *J Vasc Interv Radiol* 2004; **15**: 681–8.
3. Duszak R, Mabry MR. Clinical services in interventional radiology: results from the national Medicare database and a Society of Interventional Radiology membership survey. *J Vasc Interv Radiol* 2003; **14**: 75–81.

4. Practice Guidelines for Interventional Clinical Practice Collaborative statement from the American College of Radiology, the American Society of Interventional and Therapeutic Neuroradiology, and the Society of Interventional Radiology. *J Vasc Interv Radiol* 2005; **16**: 149–55.

5. Connolly B, Mahant S. The pediatric hospitalist and interventional radiologist: a model for clinical care in pediatric interventional radiology. *J Vasc Interv Radiol* 2006; **17**: 1733–8.

Index

Printed in the United States
by Baker & Taylor Publisher Services